POWER
OVER
PAIN

How to Get the
Pain Control You Need

■

Eric M. Chevlen, M.D.
and
Wesley J. Smith

International Task Force
Steubenville, Ohio

Library of Congress Cataloging-in-Publication Data

Chevlen, Eric M., 1949-
  Power over pain : how to get the pain control you need / Eric M. Chevlen,
    Wesley J. Smith.
  p. cm.
  ISBN 0-9710946-0-8 (trade paperback)
  1. Pain--Popular works. I. Smith, Wesley J. II. Title

  RB127 .C473 2002
  616'.0472--dc21

                                                        2001051980

Printed in the United States of America

First Edition

1 2 3 4 5 6 7 8 9 10

BOOK COVER DESIGNED BY ROXANNE LUM

To my father, Harold Chevlen...for teaching me about patients.
To my mother, Helen Chevlen...for teaching me about patience.
To my wife, Laurel Chevlen...for making my life complete.

E.M. Chevlen

To Rita Marker and Kathi Hamlon...who opened my eyes and
expanded my world.

W.J. Smith

Acknowledgements

This book would not exist without the help of many other people besides its authors. Rita Marker and Kathi Hamlon, both of the International Task Force on Euthanasia and Assisted Suicide, have been steadfast in their support, and invaluable in their editorial input. Our deep gratitude also to Bob Hiltner, Nancy Minto, Mike Marker, and John Hamlon. Purdue Pharma, L.P., gave the authors a much-appreciated unrestricted educational grant to support the creation of the book while it was still in its gestation. Our wives, Laurel and Debra, have endured years of hearing us natter about the scandal of poor pain control in America, perhaps thereby enduring some of their own. We could not have written this book without their love and support. Finally, we thank the many people with pain who have shared their frustrations and joys with us, and who provided the inspiration for this book.

■

Contents

CHAPTER 1

The Reality of Pain

This book is about pain: what causes it, how to relieve it, and equally important, how to work past the medical obstacles that too often keep patients in America from obtaining proper pain relief. It is not that we don't know how to relieve pain; it is that we simply don't get the job done. As a direct result, millions of people in this country suffer from needless pain. If you are reading this book, that probably means you or someone you love. You need relief and you need it *now*!

Untreated and under treated pain is nothing short of a national scandal. When it comes to pain control, our medical system, while certainly well intentioned, is both appallingly ineffective and obstructive, too often erecting unnecessary barriers between patients and desperately needed pain relief. That being said, this book is not primarily about changing "the system." It is about helping people who are in pain.

It is important to remember that this book cannot and does not provide a complete medical education. When you have finished reading it, you will not be qualified to hang up your medical shingle and accept patients. And while we will discuss pain-controlling strategies that are illness/condition specific, we must stress that *we are not giving you individual medical advice concerning your or your loved one's specific case*. The only person who can do that is a doctor who has examined you and who is adequately trained in the science of palliation (pain and symptom control).

It is also important to remember that, while we may mention specific brand name pain-controlling medications as examples of palliative medicine that might work in a particular circumstance, *we are not recommending these brands above others or above generics*. Nor

1

are we stating that they are the proper medicine to take in your particular circumstance. Our intent in such discussions is not to promote specific brands, but to help you help your doctor ensure that the best medical approach to controlling your pain is the one you actually receive. In other words, *please don't go to your physician asking to receive a prescription for a specific medicine based on what we write*. Instead, if you believe that a certain section of the book is relevant to your individual case, you might consider bringing it to your physician and pointing out the relevant passages as a constructive way of beginning a discussion about the best medical approach for you.

In the hope of facilitating good patient/physician communication, we will give you the information you need to discuss your pain with your doctor. We will teach you to ask the right questions. We will discuss tactics and strategies to move into more specialized pain control if initial efforts at palliation fail to provide adequate relief. In short, our purpose in writing this book is nothing less than providing you with the tools you need to be an effective pain patient in order to truly wield *power over pain*.

Pain is a word that is loosely used, so we feel the need to be quite clear about the kind of pain we are addressing. It is sometimes a metaphor—the pain of a broken heart or the pain of frustrated ambition—and sometimes used interchangeably with suffering, a related but distinct concept. Many people who have no pain at all suffer grievously, and a few people with significant pain suffer little, or, perhaps, not at all. While this book seeks to relieve suffering, it does so primarily in the context of reducing the experience of physical pain.

Defining Pain

There are several highly technical definitions of pain that appear in medical textbooks. They describe, in the precise and arcane language so beloved by doctors and scientists, the exact technical meaning

2

of the term "pain," and the many fine distinctions between it and related terms. We could quote them to you, but we won't: your eyes would only glaze over, and you would stop reading. What matters to us—and we presume to you, the reader—are not academic definitions, but rather a recognition of the dreadful reality that pain makes of daily experience, and, more importantly, what can be done to relieve your suffering. Indeed, that is our purpose and our deepest desire. Still, we have to reach a common understanding of what it is we are writing about, and that requires us to take a few pages to define our subject.

The International Association for the Study of Pain is the major world scientific body engaged in combating pain in all its manifestations. It defines pain as "an unpleasant sensory and emotional experience associated with actual or potential tissue damage, or described in terms of such damage." This definition is certainly short and accurate, and provides us with key concepts that are necessary to understand if we are to comprehend why it hurts and what can be done to make it stop hurting.

Notice first that pain is described as a "sensory" experience. This means that pain is *by definition* something *you feel* rather than something that is measured by your doctor or other medical professional. That is one reason why some people in pain find it difficult to get their doctors to take their pain seriously. It is a subjective rather than an objective phenomenon.

This makes pain hard to measure. X-rays may show broken bones or pinched nerves, but they do not show pain. Blood tests, CT scans and MRIs can reveal the presence of disease or injury, but they do not show pain. There is no thermometer to measure pain, no cuff that can be applied to a sore arm to tell the doctor how much it hurts. There is no device we can use to tell us whether or not a person is experiencing any pain at all. In fact, doctors often report seeing patients whose x-rays reveal numerous cancer tumors, yet these patients repeatedly deny having the least bit of pain.

On the other hand, patients may be completely disabled by agonizing pain from injuries that are either invisible or show the most trivial damage using even the most sophisticated medical imaging device. Thus, while experience might lead us to reasonably anticipate that specific injuries or illnesses will produce expected levels of pain, that does not mean it will necessarily happen. The same abnormality on imaging studies may be associated in one person with an agony requiring intensive treatment with the strongest medicines, and in another with a mild ache treatable with mere aspirin or Tylenol®. Pain is an individual experience, and wise doctors always approach it as such.

 ## *From the Doctor's Journal:*

I often lecture to my colleagues around the country concerning pain and its management. As is expected on such occasions, I begin my lecture with the formal, precise, scientific definition of pain. But there is a mischievous part of me that is dissatisfied with such a lecture and such a definition. Rather than give them my usual formal presentation, I'm tempted to substitute a simple demonstration for the academic lecture. Instead of words, I'm tempted to simply place a box of gravel at the entrance to the lecture hall. In my imagination, I instruct my audience members to take a piece of gravel, just a single, tiny pebble, and place it in one of their shoes. Then they are to walk around all day with that single pebble beneath the soles of their feet. They are to feel that tiny stone digging into their soles with every step, and feel it dig in with more force when they walk a little faster or climb stairs. They are to feel those mere tiny stones when they stand in an elevator, and dread when the elevator stops its descent with a bump that seems gentle to everyone else, but torturous to them. They are to feel those tiny, lone

4

pebbles grow in their feet, to swell in their effects, until they feel like cracked bayonets beneath their feet. And their single pebbles are not to be removed all day.

By the end of the day of my imaginary instruction, the practical experience of walking with a tiny pebble in one shoe would give each audience member a far better understanding of the reality of chronic pain than would my usual lecture. I would hope that my audience would realize that if they're so miserably uncomfortable from a simple little pebble in a shoe, how much more suffering must be the daily experiences of those whose pain is not so easily relieved. How much more must be the suffering of those whose pain brings them to a doctor's office in the first place. Yes, the textbook definition of pain is important, but far more important to my professional audience is to get at least a peek into the life of those in chronic pain. Trying to understand pain without a heart of compassion and without belief in its subjective reality is like trying to understand a love letter from a chemical analysis of its ink.

Because the individual experience of pain varies widely and is essentially not measurable, it can be a very clever foe, particularly if patients do not effectively communicate to their doctor what they are feeling, or if their doctor discounts the patient's description of pain. What is the implication of this? This point is fundamental: *effective pain diagnosis and control require effective communication.* The patient must be able to communicate to the doctor what the pain feels like, its severity, its quality (sharp, dull, etc.), when it hurts and when it doesn't, and its duration. At the same time, doctors need to be open to their patients' communication, however expressed, and try to understand exactly what it is that the patient feels. Furthermore, since patients often act as if "good patients" don't "bother" their doctors with complaints about pain, diligent physicians know that they should walk the extra mile to draw out information from their patients about pain.

Unfortunately, our medical system is not geared toward taking pain seriously. Do you doubt this? Come with us on a tour of a hospital intensive care unit. There we find the patient lying on his back in bed, a bevy of tubes running in and out of every orifice. The electrocardiograph monitor displays every heartbeat. An arterial line measures blood pressure second-by-second. On the patient's finger is a transcutaneous probe that tells us at a glance how well saturated the blood is with oxygen. Why, there's enough hi-tech medicine just monitoring the patient's condition that you'd think you were in the cockpit of a jet plane.

Now, let's visit a typical hospital ward. On the bedside hospital chart we find daily or more frequent measurements of the patient's serum sodium, potassium, glucose, and chloride. The patient's temperature, food intake, urinary output, and even bowel movements are measured with precision, and they are recorded on the chart, as are the daily examination of lungs, abdomen, and other vital organs. Not only are all these factors weighed, measured, and recorded, but also the records of these measurements are kept permanently, first in the overflowing medical records department, and later on microfilm. The microfilm is treated like a national treasure, stored in temperature-controlled caves, safe from damage by sun, rain, and even nuclear attack.

Yet, for all of the millions of dollars devoted to storing all of this medical information about each and every patient, *few, if any, observations are made or records kept about whether the patient was in pain.* Most hospital charts make no mention of the health factor that is often of the greatest importance to the patient—his or her level of pain—and the adequacy of treatment efforts to control it. This is a telling omission that speaks volumes about the relative unimportance historically given to controlling pain in clinical medicine.

Happily, medicine is beginning to change its tune. A movement has emerged within the profession to refer to pain as the "fifth vital sign." The idea is to recognize that measurement of pain is as important to the patient's well-being as measuring temperature, pulse, respiration, and blood pressure, and that controlling pain is as important as maintaining 120/80 blood pressure and healthy levels of cholesterol. The symbolic importance alone of charting pain should do much in coming years to help focus medicine on the important goal of reducing pain and misery.

This is no small matter. The proper treatment of pain is as important to the patient's welfare as is treating other forms of ill health. It is important for its own sake, of course. Nothing feels "better" than the absence of pain after a period of significant suffering, as anyone who has ever suffered more than fleeting pain will tell you. It is also important for the sake of the patient's family, since pain can significantly distort the sufferer's personality, making the patient irritable, impatient, hostile, or depressed, and potentially rending the fabric of intimate and familial relationships. Pain also impacts the workplace, causing absences, making people less productive, less able to work with others, and less able to attend to the tasks at hand. In fact, pain is estimated to cause 50 million lost work days each year, costing employers more than $3 billion in wages paid to employees unable to work.

Beyond these immediate benefits of controlling pain, there is evidence from animal experiments that the proper management of pain can actually prolong life. Animals in pain seem to have impaired immune systems; they are at greater risk of dying from infections and even cancers. It is likely that proper treatment of pain does more than just enhance the quality of life. It may even increase its quantity. Yes, pain truly is the fifth vital sign.

From the Doctor's Journal:

As we are writing this book, there is a young woman under my care for severe left arm pain. The name of her disease is complex regional pain syndrome (CRPS). She has suffered from it for about a year. Although her pain and ability to do daily activities have improved dramatically in the past few weeks of treatment, the pain is not yet as well managed as I expect it will be with further modification of therapy. Periodically, she gets an injection of lidocaine, a local anesthetic, in the nerves in her neck that go to her arm. That gives her complete, although temporary, relief of her pain.

She pays a price for this relief: temporary paralysis of the arm. She calls it "the wet noodle" effect. I asked her once whether she would accept permanent pain relief at the price of permanent paralysis. It was a theoretical question, both because that cannot be accomplished, and because there will be ways of controlling her pain far short of such a drastic solution. But she smiled at me and said, "Get rid of this pain permanently and have a paralyzed arm? I'd do it in a heartbeat!" A friend of hers, who was with her in the office, also with CRPS, nodded in understanding and agreement. I knew that they were not exaggerating, that they were perfectly sincere. They would rather have a paralyzed limb than one in severe chronic pain. That brief exchange reinforced in my mind the horror of living in chronic pain, and the importance of taking the patient's complaints seriously.

Still, because pain is not measurable, and can't be seen, smelled, heard, or touched, the complaints of pain sufferers are often discounted or even disbelieved by their families and doctors when they describe how much they hurt. Imagine the agony of being disbelieved that you are in agony! For years you may have lived a responsible life as a parent, a spouse, a worker, a volunteer, a church/synagogue/mosque member. Now, because of pain you can no longer work, and barely get through the day. As for hobbies and avocations you once enjoyed—forget about it! Golf? You can hardly swing the club. Gardening? You can barely stoop over, let alone pull weeds and plant flowers for any length of time. Sex with your spouse? Not likely! Who can enjoy intimacy when just being touched hurts so much. Travel? Vacations would be a waste of money. Your external sources of self-esteem have been utterly gutted. You are miserable. In your darkest moments, you may even contemplate suicide.

So, you go to doctor after doctor asking for, and later even begging for, relief. Again and again, you sit in a generic waiting room, looking at the same *National Geographic* magazine from five years ago, but not really reading the words or absorbing the pictures. Finally, you are called into a cramped examining room where you are told to get into a skimpy gown and sit on the table covered by what seems to be an oversized roll of paper from the delicatessen. There you wait . . . and wait . . . and wait some more. The doctor finally comes in, gives you the once over, and quickly tunes out as you tell your tale of woe. You can almost see it on the doctor's face: "Nah, this guy's not for real." The frustration seethes within you. Why on earth would you endure this abuse— often at considerable expense— if you weren't in pain? The very fact that you are there despite all the inconveniences, cost, and often humiliation is testimony of the harsh reality of your complaint. The time has come for doctors to see such histories as evidence of sincerity and suffering, not of emotional instability.

From the Doctor's Journal:

Not too long ago I was treating a young man whose life had been ruined by unrelieved back pain. He had injured his back on the job, and gone through the usual hassles associated with the Worker's Compensation system to get payment for the treatment of his back pain. His x-rays were unimpressive, revealing nothing terribly out of the ordinary. Still, his suffering was enormous. He was unemployed, unemployable, socially isolated, and besieged by a feeling of utter hopelessness. Yet, his previous doctors had not believed he hurt as badly as he claimed.

He came into the office one day wincing more than usual, and walking more stiffly than was his norm. When I examined his back, I noticed that along his spine was a line of angry-looking red welts. "Good heavens, what happened?" I asked him. He told me that he had heard from a friend (God protect us all from such friends!) that a man in a nearby town was curing multiple sclerosis by the application of bee stings. He reasoned that since chronic pain, like multiple sclerosis, was a neurological disorder, perhaps the bee stings might help his pain, too. Neither my patient nor his friend recognized the man for what he was—a dangerous charlatan. Of course this bee sting "therapy" had only added to his pain, and no doubt to his shame as well.

At first I thought, "What lunacy to stick bees on a sore back!" But then I considered the matter more deeply, and I saw the bee sting episode not as an exercise in self-abuse or therapeutic sabotage, but as an expression of absolute desperation. My patient had reached the point of believing (wrongly, as it turned out) that his pain was already so bad that literally nothing could make it worse. He was willing to try anything to rid himself of the accursed pain. And this was a man whom many doctors had thought was simply exaggerating. He wasn't, and the bee sting episode proved it.

■

Why Different People Feel Pain Differently

When people talk about pain, they often speak imprecisely of their "pain threshold." Outside of a pain research laboratory, this is a questionable concept at best. It confuses pain with the stimulus that causes the sensation that is felt. Here's a simple illustration: Ted, Bill, and Jim are boys playing a game of tag in which the one who is slapped on the back is "it." All three are not wearing shirts. The boys run and play, giggle and laugh. Jim, the first "it," finally catches up to Ted, and slaps him solidly on the back with a loud "smack." The slap is a *stimulus*. The *sensation* that the slap created is mild pain. Ted barely flinches, and the game continues. Being "it," he now chases down Bill and delivers a slap of equal force. However, Bill has a nasty sunburn on his back, and thus he feels more pain from the same stimulus. In this case, the slap elicits a loud yelp. The game continues, and Bill chases down Jim, giving him another slap of equal intensity. Two days before, Jim had fallen off his bike and badly scraped his back right where the Bill's slap hits. "OWWWW!" he screams at the top of his voice, as tears begin to flow.

For purposes of the illustration, the three boys had different physical conditions, resulting in different levels of complaining from the same force applied by the slaps. Remember, this was only an illustration. People complain of different levels of pain even when they do not have any obvious differences in their health. Some people just report feeling more pain than others report. It is not simply a matter of "pain threshold" or a person's character or lack thereof, or of strength or weakness. Purely and simply, the same stimulus can cause different people to experience different levels of pain.

We see proof of this in animal studies. In animals there is an enormous variation in pain-related behavior when a uniform stimulus is applied. (Remember, we cannot ask the animals about their pain, we can only measure their behavior.) We have no reason to think that there are differences in character among laboratory mice ("Gee, that Larry in cage 12 is a real wimp!") to account for these differences. Rather, we know that the central nervous systems of these animals act differently, causing pain-related signals to increase or decrease from the site of the pain stimulus to the brain, which translates those signals into the sensation of pain. It is not that these animals tolerate the same pain differently. Like Jim, Ted, and Bill, we presume that *they actually experience different levels of pain* from the same stimulus.

It is as if we wanted to compare, say, the bird-carrying capability of two people, but asked one to carry a sparrow and the other to carry an ostrich. We would not say that they have different "bird-carrying thresholds," but rather that they are carrying very different birds. The same is true of pain, but they are invisible birds. The pain one person feels from a stimulus may be a sparrow, and for his best friend, an ostrich. That is why communication is so important. It is up to the patient to tell the doctor how heavy a load of pain he or she is carrying. Doctors have no independent way knowing.

Pain Is an Emotional Experience

So far we have described pain as a physical occurrence. But it is more than that. It is also an emotional experience.

From the Doctor's Journal:

I entered the field of pain medicine after many years of practicing medical oncology (cancer medicine). I was certainly used to treating patients who were having crises in their lives. The cancer patients expressed the usual range of emotion I would expect for someone in that circumstance, ranging from courage and stoicism to anguish. But, frankly, the emotional aspect was not the dominant one.

In contrast, virtually all of my pain patients were emotional about their affliction in a way I was not then used to, and which, when I was green in the field of pain medicine, used to annoy me. I was actually a bit intolerant. I used to think that the practice of pain medicine would be a lot more fun if the patients were just less emotional about it. Later I realized that my wanting pain patients to be unemotional was like an obstetrician wanting to practice his specialty, but not wanting to deal with pregnant women. Emotions and pain go hand-in-hand.

We are, so to speak, hard-wired to experience emotion as part of the experience of pain. The reason for this, again, is basic physiology. As most people learn in high school biology classes, pain is experienced when the "pain information" moves from the site of the painful stimulus, via nerves to the spinal cord, which ships it up into the brain. What they do not know is that the part of the brain designated to first receive the pain information is also the part that controls emotion. Thus we not only "feel" pain physically, we also "feel" it emotionally. We can no more suppress these emotions than we can choose to see in black and white rather than color. It's just not in our physiological cards.

Different types of pain generally create differing emotions in the patient. People suffering from acute pain (pain of short duration) usually feel anxious. Think of the late middle-aged smoker who has a squeezing chest pain radiating to his jaw and left arm. His anxiety is not merely because he believes (most likely, correctly) that he is having a heart attack. *The pain itself induces the anxiety.* The unlucky patient who is passing her fourth kidney stone knows the whole painful routine by heart, knows that she is unlikely to die or become seriously incapacitated, but still experiences anxiety along with the pain.

This isn't by accident. Pain is one of the body's most important protective mechanisms, allowing us to recognize and withdraw from dangerous situations. The emotions associated with the pain have assisted, at least throughout human prehistory and until the modern era, with this protective function. Imagine one of our cave-dwelling ancestors who has an unhappy encounter in the dark with a bear. When the bear slashes him with its claws, his anxiety, partially caused by the pain of his wound, is wonderfully useful. He knows, or more accurately he *feels*, that he is in a dangerous situation, even if he can't see the bear in the darkness of the cave. He doesn't stop to ponder what could have caused the sudden pain across his back. He reacts immediately and runs away as fast as his legs will move him. In this situation, anxiety is a very protective emotion.

In contrast to acute pain, the emotion associated with chronic (long-lasting) pain is usually depression. Again, this has often had a protective benefit. If the caveman had his arm broken by the bear, but miraculously survived the attack, he would doubtless have pain for several months while the broken bone healed. The depression associated with this pain would actually be useful. A depressed person is not an adventurous one. Our caveman will sit quietly and morosely in the back of his cave while his arm heals. That's a far better way to allow healing than going out in brisk new bear-encountering adventures. Pain-induced depression is the body's way of saying, "Take it easy for a while."

14

Nowadays, of course, the depression that accompanies chronic pain seldom has this protective benefit. We no longer live in caves, and few of us encounter bears on the way to the supermarket. The depression caused by pain merely adds to its misery.

Unfortunately, the unwary physician may completely misinterpret the coexistence of depression with pain. If he cannot find a cause for pain, the doctor is apt to conclude that the depression is the cause of the pain, rather than vice versa. While treating depression may facilitate the treatment of the pain, treating only the depression does not "cure" the patient of chronic pain. On the other hand, successful treatment of pain often kills two birds with one stone— the pain and the depression.

 From the Doctor's Journal:

The depression associated with chronic pain may be severe, and such cases may warrant a combined treatment aimed at both aspects of the patient's suffering. One of my patients became despondent when, after eight months of successful treatment of chronic severe low back pain, he had a temporary setback. He had had about fifteen years of misery before his remission, and he feared that the remission would prove to be merely a tiny oasis in the bleak desert of his painful life. His wife reported that he had said to her, "Maybe cousin Raymond had the right answer." I learned that cousin Raymond, too, had had chronic back pain, but had never seen a pain specialist. His pain ended only when he shot himself. Happily, with treatment for his depression as well as his pain, my patient was able to get past his depression and got on with his life.

Let's return one last time to the definition of pain: an unpleasant sensory and emotional experience associated with actual or potential tissue damage (injury), or described in terms of such damage. It is important to emphasize that *actual tissue damage, such as that found in arthritis, burns, or cancer, need not be present* for the patient to experience pain. Pain is present simply on the basis of its honest description, such as when the patient describes the pain experience as burning, squeezing, tearing, stabbing, etc. Normal physical examinations, normal x-rays and normal blood tests do not rule out the presence of pain. Indeed, pain is often the most frustrating for both patient and doctor when the cause cannot be discovered. It cannot be repeated often enough: the doctor's failure to find the cause of pain does not mean the pain originates "in the patient's head."

Here's an example that may help clarify any misunderstanding. Imagine that there are two women standing before you, each one saying, "My feet feel like they're in boiling-hot water." On further inspection, you see that in fact one of them *does* have her feet immersed in boiling-hot water. The origin and validity of her complaint are self-evident. But the other woman's feet are not in hot water. They're not in water at all. The origin of her complaint is not self-evident. You examine her feet, and all seems normal. Just as you are concluding that she is a hypochondriac, you notice a bottle of insulin in her pocket. Suddenly, you realize that she is a diabetic and conclude that her pain is as real as is the woman's whose feet are being boiled. The nerves of the woman standing in hot water are sending signals from a real noxious (tissue-damaging) stimulus. The diabetic's damaged nerves in her feet are sending "false" pain signals that are virtually identical to the type of message that would be sent if her feet really were in hot water. *This doesn't mean her pain is false. It is very real!*

No matter how your pain originates or even if its origin cannot be found, if you are feeling the unpleasant physical and emotional experience associated with actual or potential tissue damage (or described in terms of such damage), you are, by definition, in pain.

Measuring Pain

Despite the fact that pain is entirely a subjective experience, it can be measured and assessed with the help of the patient. By asking the patient on repeated occasions to describe the severity of his or her pain, and by using a standardized way of asking that question, the doctor can have a reproducible measurement of the pain's severity.

There are several different ways of asking this question. One way is to ask the patient to describe the pain as "mild, moderate, or severe." Another way is to ask the patient to describe the severity of the pain on a scale of 0 to 10, with 0 indicating no pain at all, and 10 indicating pain as bad as one can imagine it being. Yet another way is to present the patient with a horizontal line, about six inches in length. One end of the line is marked "no pain" and the other end is marked "pain as bad as it can be." The patient is instructed to make a vertical hash mark through the line indicating where to place his level of pain on the no pain/pain scale. The distance from the "no pain" end to the vertical hash mark is measured in millimeters, and that number then reflects the pain as measured on a 0 to 100 scale.

There are even tools to measure a child's pain. The child in pain is presented with a series of pictured faces, ranging from one with a broad smile to one with a down-turned frown and tears rolling down the cheeks. He's asked to select the face that is the best picture of how he feels.

It bears emphasis that the pain score derived from the procedure described above can be used to compare pain intensities at different times for the same person, but not between people. It is meaningless to say that, because Bill scores his pain as an 8 and Sarah scores hers as a 7, Bill's pain is greater than Sarah's. It is equally meaningless to compare pain between people because different people can never experience the same pain. The pain score is useful only to see how Bill's or Sarah's pain changes over time, for example, before and after treatment.

The misconception that we can compare pain between people is deeply ingrained. We can see two people exposed to the same stimulus, such as a slap on the back or an operative procedure, and we illogically assume that their pain is or ought to be identical. But pain, by its nature, is something that cannot be compared between people. It is entirely subjective.

Imagine two people standing before you, scratching their noses. Each one says his nose is itchy. They then begin to argue as to whose nose is itchier. The first one accuses the other of scratching his nose far more than his itchiness warrants. The second accuses the first of having a low threshold for itchiness. The argument is laughable, of course, because it is completely meaningless to compare itching between people. Until people grow two noses, they will never be able to know the itchiness of more than one. Similarly, we can never really know the pain experienced by another.

Pain is subjective, but it is measurable. That measurement allows us to know how badly people hurt based on their own perceptions and on whether our treatment attempts are working. Frankly, it is not terribly important which tool the physician uses to measure pain, but it is vital that it be measured. Unmeasured pain is likely to be untreated or undertreated pain.

Now that we understand what pain is, how different people experience it differently, and how it cannot be seen but can be measured, we will explore the mechanisms that allow us to experience—and to decrease the experience of—pain.

CHAPTER 2

—■—

How We Feel Pain

Pain is one of the great banes of human life. Paradoxically, it is also one of our most vital defense systems, the proper working of which is essential for a long and healthy life.

If you doubt this, consider the rare, tragic cases of children born without the ability to sense pain. Most of them become severely disabled in childhood because of repeated untended injuries. They are completely unaware of them because they do not possess a "pain warning siren." Similarly, patients afflicted with leprosy suffer progressive mutilation of their extremities, not due to the ravages of the disease itself, but rather because the disease destroys the ability to sense pain in the affected limbs. People who have spinal cord damage must also pay special attention to the physical state of their bodies. They are unable to feel discomfort from prolonged sitting or lying in one position. Because of that, they may develop bedsores, which can progress to deep ulcers all the way down to the bone. Like the patients with leprosy or congenital absence of pain sensation, they lack the often-mixed blessing of pain.

Sensing pain is one of our primary defenses against significant injury. It is what allows us to reflexively pull our hand off the hot stove without needing to hear the "sizzle" to warn us that what's cooking isn't bacon. Even chronic pain, for all its misery, has its beneficial uses. In ages past, when many bouts of chronic pain were probably due to reversible injuries, it had the especially protective effect of deterring reinjury, thereby promoting healing. Today, most chronic pain has little biological benefit. The person with rheumatoid arthritis, or migraine, or cancer receives no survival value from suffering pain. On the contrary, the ongoing agony significantly diminishes the quality of life, and may even shorten it. In such cases, the relief of pain is more than a humanitarian exercise. In a metaphorical, but only slightly exaggerated, sense, relief of severe chronic pain restores the living dead to renewed vigor and life.

 From the Doctor's Journal:

It is often said that it is difficult to describe great pain to someone who has not experienced it. The same is true of pain relief. I have noticed how very often my patients reflect a near-desperate urgency in their need to express the difference they have come to experience in their lives after they have achieved successful and sustained pain relief. Like the Ancient Mariner of Coleridge's poem, they seem compelled to explain the weird pain voyage that they, alone, have traveled, the horrific country they visited, and from which, at long last, they have returned. In their gratitude and relief, they often confuse the agent with the cause. The most common expression I hear from them is this: "Dr. Chevlen, you've given me my life back."

I used to dismiss this in my mind as hyperbole, but I have come to realize that, in fact, there is a deep truth in their description of what has been restored. I remember reading in the Talmud that a person in severe pain must be treated with the same special regard as one suffering from a potentially fatal illness. Just as almost all the laws of the Torah may be set aside, if necessary, to save a life, they may also be set aside to relieve severe pain. The sages of the Talmud knew what it has taken me twenty years of practice to learn, that a life lived in intractable pain is not a full life.

20

> In a way, relieving intractable pain is like saving a life, and saving one life has been compared to saving the whole world. So, when I come home and my wife asks me how my day at the office was, I tell her that I saved the whole world today. "That's nice, dear," she says. "Did you remember to take out the garbage?" Apparently she, at least, has no difficulty in distinguishing the agent from the cause.

The pain system is fascinatingly, and sometimes frustratingly, complex. Indeed, there isn't just "one" way that the body regulates pain; it turns out that there are many. Moreover, scientists still don't understand pain fully, and are working hard to unlock the secrets of this long-neglected area of physiology.

This is an important enterprise. An army needs intelligence agents to inform it of the strength and deployment of the enemy. Similarly, if we want to have power over pain, if we want to vanquish this ancient enemy, we must first understand it. By learning about the normal ways in which pain works and the manner in which the body and mind react to it, we shall learn how we can manipulate the many bodily systems involved in feeling pain, so as to relieve or even eliminate the sensation entirely when its presence is harmful to our well-being.

Nerve Fibers: The Cells That Sense Pain

Pain happens: a child falls and scrapes her knee; a man is shot during a robbery; cancer invades the normal tissues of an elderly woman's abdomen; arthritis prevents the trout fisherman from making his own flies. Under normal conditions, when there is a potentially damaging force applied to the body—the scraped knee, the bullet, the cancer, the swelling of the joints—pain fibers embedded in the affected tissues ring a warning alarm. This is the pain stimulus or, to put it another way, the beginning of the pain signal. From the site of trauma or disease, the signal then races toward the spinal cord along remarkable single-cell nerve fibers that have the biological task of sending such pain-related information to the central nervous system.

Because the perception of pain is so important, injury-sensing nerve fibers are located throughout virtually the entire body. Curiously, the brain itself is the only major organ that lacks the ability to perceive pain. However, as anyone who has had the terrible headache of meningitis will tell you, the meninges (the lining of the brain) is certainly richly endowed with pain fibers.

In order to better understand the pain transmission system, think of these nerve fibers heading toward the spinal cord as akin to the individual lines which make up a telephone cable. Just as the lines from each home join together as individual parts of a more complex high-tech cable headed toward the telephone switching station, so the nerves from many sites within the body merge together into a larger nerve headed toward the spinal cord.

It is important to note that this "cable" of nerves is not a one-way street. Nor is it restricted to carrying pain information alone. In addition to the abundance of sensory information, such as pain, heat, cold, itching, limb position, etc., headed toward the spinal cord, there is also a significant amount of outbound information going through this "cable." Some of the outbound information is under conscious control, such as the signals that tell the many muscles of the forearm to swat a mosquito, or caress a child's head. Other outbound as well as inbound signals are not under conscious control. They obey, so to speak, their own laws, and thus are called the autonomic ("self law") nervous system.

The autonomic nervous system controls body activities such as sweating, dilatation of blood vessels, and even goosebumps. The autonomic nervous system within the chest and abdomen controls, among other things, dilatation of the airways, heart rate, and the action of the digestive system. With so much back-and-forth nerve activity going on, do the outbound and inbound signals ever get crossed? Absolutely. Sometimes injury or disease may cause a misconnection between the outbound autonomic information and the inbound pain signal. Every time the message leaves the spinal cord telling the skin to sweat, for example, the misconnection can lead to a turnaround, and become an inbound signal which would then be perceived by the brain as pain, just as if there had been actual tissue injury. This can lead to self-perpetuating pain: pain often causes anxiety, which in turn, causes sweating, leading to pain, leading to anxiety. Talk about a vicious circle!

In fact, this dismal scenario is theorized to be part of the mechanism of the painful condition formerly known as "reflex sympathetic dystrophy." This rare, painful condition was first described in the medical literature in the 19th century, and it was called causalgia. Its modern name is complex regional pain syndrome (CRPS). In its major form, it may follow significant injury to one of the nerves of the limbs. However, even relatively minor trauma, for reasons yet unknown, can occasionally precipitate this pain. Those who have it describe it as a uniquely painful experience. Compounding the suffering of the patients with CRPS is the fact that this interaction of the autonomic and pain systems cannot be "seen" by any known testing method. This makes diagnosis difficult, and, tragically, often leads ignorant clinicians to doubt the severity or even the presence of the patient's pain complaints.

But we digress. Once the pain receptor cells are stimulated from whatever the source, the resulting pain "signals" are transmitted electrically toward the spinal cord. Yes, electrically. There is an actual current flowing through each pain receptor cell toward the spinal cord. Each of the pain receptor cells—the same cells that are bundled together along with other inbound and outbound nerve fibers—stretches from its ending to the spinal cord. So, if you stub your toe, the information about that trauma travels along a number of living cables of cells that were stimulated by the toe hitting the rock. Each of these fibers is one cell that is as long as the length from the end of your toe to where the fiber ends at the lower portion of the spinal cord—perhaps three feet long or more, depending on your height. Other nerve fibers will be short or long, depending on where they are in the body and where in the spinal cord they communicate their information. What remarkable biological engineering!

Sensing Pain Through Chemistry

It takes a fraction of a second for the signal to reach the end of the nerve fiber at the spinal cord. From here, the pain transmission system shifts to a different mode of communication, because the nerve fiber that is stimulated to carry the pain message does not connect electrically with the spinal cord. There is a microscopic gap at the junction in the spinal cord where the first pain nerve cell meets the next nerve cell that accepts the pain information and begins the process of moving it along toward the brain. This gap between nerves is called a synapse.

The lack of contact between the nerve cells stymies the electric current, since, for pain to be communicated up the spinal cord toward the brain electrically, the membranes of the nerves would have to be touching. Even though the space between the membranes is only an incredibly tiny 20 millionths of a millimeter, that would still be enough to stop the pain signal—except for the miracle of chemistry. As it is, the nerves use chemical communication methods to pass along the pain message originally brought to the spinal cord electrically by the nerve fibers.

Here's how it works. At the end of the nerve fiber and every spinal cord nerve cell, there is a pre-packaged supply of chemical messengers contained in little bubbles called vesicles. When the

24

electrical signal reaches the end of the first pain nerve fiber, the vesicle merges with the nerve membrane, and its contents are emptied into the synaptic cleft (the space between the nerves). The chemicals then quickly cross the tiny distance to the other side of the cleft, triggering an electrical impulse in the next nerve. This electrical pulse shoots through the second nerve, and causes release of its vesicles at the other end. Their contents bridge the next synaptic cleft, stimulating another electrical response in the next nerve, and so on. By the end of the second nerve, the signal has reached the base of the brain. Of course, most of the nerves don't connect with simply one other nerve. Each one has multiple synapses, and each of these in turn has multiple synapses. It's easy to see how this spreading wave of information can incorporate the activity of millions of nerve cells. All of this, of course, happens in less than a second.

Changing from a solely electrical to a chemical/electrical communication allows a far more sophisticated pain message to be sent to the brain than would otherwise be the case. Why? It appears that the vesicles in different nerve endings may hold different chemical signals, making it likely that a different chemical signal is sent for different degrees of pain. For example, there is some evidence that the chemical called "substance P" (yes, that's "P" for "pain") is a key signal in severe pain, while other chemicals deliver the signal for mild and moderate pain. This permits nuance and differentiation in the perception of pain. In other words, you can tell pain caused by a burn, from that caused by a punch, from that caused by a pinprick.

The chemistry of pain transmission provides some wonderful opportunities for exercising power over pain. A quick example of this will suffice for now. Everyone has heard stories of soldiers shot in battle who continue to fight, often unaware of the severity of their wounds. They later claim that, in fact, they felt no pain, or

25

only a trivial amount, from their serious wounds. These stories are usually used to exemplify the courage of the soldiers. Courageous though they were, these stories of not feeling pain are not evidence of their courage. (Courage is duty performed despite fear, and is independent of whether an injury is actually sustained.) Why? When the soldiers say that they felt no pain, they are telling the literal truth. It is not that they felt pain and persevered (that, too, occurs in battle, but is not the subject of this discussion). They really felt no pain.

But how can that be? The body has a natural pain controlling mechanism to dampen the pain signals before they reach the centers of the brain that consciously perceive them. One of the important sites of that mechanism is the spinal cord. There are nerves descending from the brain, down the spinal cord, which have direct and indirect synapse communication with neurons that send pain messages up the spinal cord to the brain. These descending nerves secrete a chemical that dampens the pain signal being sent up the cord. Similar pain-suppressing cell systems are found in sites along the pain pathway in the brain. These chemicals diminish pain in the same way that morphine does, and this explains the name of one of these natural analgesic (painkilling) chemicals, endorphin (from "endogenous morphine").

The place where the endorphin and related natural chemicals bind is called the opioid receptor. (An opioid is a narcotic.) It is also the place where morphine and similar narcotics act. When the opioid receptor is stimulated, whether naturally by bodily substances like endorphin or from taking morphine or similar synthetic agents, the body's ability to transmit pain information is interfered with. Thus, what the body does naturally when faced with overwhelming painful stimulation, we do artificially with morphine and other medicines— bringing great relief from searing, agonizing pain. The details of how these drugs work and the types of illnesses and conditions for which they relieve pain will be discussed in another chapter.

The Pain Is in Your Head

Without the brain, these chemical signals would be like the proverbial tree that fell in a forest but made no sound. Just as it takes a brain to interpret the sound waves of the fallen tree into the perception of noise, so it takes a brain to translate the chemical signals sent through the nervous system into the sensation we know as pain.

Here is how that process works. When the signal has climbed the spinal cord and arrives in the brain, it is split into different parts. The first brain way station in the path of pain perception is the thalamus, a part of the brain deeply involved with, among other things, the experience of emotion. As we mentioned before and will again, this is probably one reason why pain and emotions are so extensively interconnected.

But the thalamus is only part of the story. Because each of the nerve cells has multiple synapses, the transmission of the pain message acts like a savings account enjoying compound interest—the signals multiply as they are passed from nerve to nerve, leaving plenty of sensation to go around in the brain. Beyond the thalamus, the pain signal is also transmitted to other parts of the brain: a section that "perceives" location and an area that provides meaning to what is being experienced. In this way, pain not only is felt as a sensation, but the brain informs the comprehending mind where it hurts, perhaps why it hurts, and whether the pain is cause for alarm.

It is easy to see why all of these perceptions about pain are important. You touch a hot stove. Almost instantly you pull your hand away, even before you are aware of pain. Why is that? One of the connections of the pain nerve fibers in the spinal cord is to the muscles that cause withdrawal of the hand. This withdrawal from a harmful stimulus is built deeply into the body's mechanism. It can be seen even in people who have a severed spinal cord as well as in animals whose brains (or a major part of them) have been removed. Within a second or so, as your brain consciously participates in the experience of the burning sensation, your mind recognizes that the pain is in your hand, and informs you that the cause of pain is not life threatening. Alternatively, you feel a sudden, severe pain in your chest that feels like an elephant sitting on you, accompanied by a shooting pain down your left arm. The brain not only mediates the feeling of the different sensations of pain, but also makes you aware that this is no small matter, causing you to reach for the phone to dial 911.

In many ways, of course, this explanation is extremely simplified, if not outright glib. After all, how is it possible that this squishy stuff we call the brain can cause such differences in our sense of awareness? Does the brain, in fact, "cause" consciousness or is it merely a necessary instrument for it? Can we have consciousness without a brain? Many religious traditions teach that we can; they call it a soul. The interaction of mind and brain (to say nothing of souls, minds, and brains) is a deep mystery, known in the classical philosophy literature as the mind-body problem, but more recently as the consciousness problem. But other than perhaps causing a headache, we need not worry about such issues. This, after all, is a practical book, not a philosophical treatise.

For now, suffice it to say that awareness of the existence of pain, as well as its location and implication, is perceived by millions of cells distributed widely throughout the brain. There is no little man sitting on a stool in the cerebrum beneath a sign labeled "the ouch stops here." By understanding how pain is received by the body, communicated to the brain, and perceived in the brain, science has been able to develop very effective medical techniques to trick the body into feeling no or little pain where extreme pain should exist.

The most serious problem people have in getting relief from pain isn't in the area of how to do it—we pretty much know that. It is in making sure the job gets done. Without a doubt, access to effective treatment is too often the biggest pain control problem of all.

CHAPTER 3

How Do You Spell Relief?
N-S-A-I-D

The biological workings of the pain pathway are such that signals sent by the nerves, through the spinal cord, to the brain can be modified in much the same way that a stereo CD player's bass can be adjusted. Only, instead of better sound, you feel relief from pain.

To see how this works, let's start at the site of the injury or illness. That's where the pain signal originates and where the sensitivity of the pain fiber—that is, its irritability—is sometimes increased by chemicals that are present at the site. These chemicals can be real rascals. They make up a witches' brew that causes the heat, redness, soreness, and loss of function associated with inflammation, commonly known as swelling.

So why do we have these chemicals? Look at what happens when an injury occurs. Blood flow increases, bringing in more white cells to fight infection—a definite benefit. Then blood vessels become more porous, making it easier for white cells and antibodies to seep out of the blood vessels into the injured tissue. It is this increased leaking of fluid that causes swelling. The accompanying tenderness and loss of function is what causes the person to "baby" the sore spot, reducing the risk of further injury—another definite benefit.

The mixture of the chemicals that causes swelling has been called an "inflammatory soup." One of the "soup's" ingredients is a member of the class of chemicals called prostaglandins. The prostaglandin found at the site of inflammation actually changes the function of the nerve fiber there. It lowers the threshold for the cell's electrical discharge. That electrical discharge, you will recall, is the first step toward the perception of pain.

What does "lowering the threshold" mean? It means that the affected nerve cells become like hair triggers. It takes less force or trauma to make the pain nerve fiber discharge and send a signal to the spinal cord. The technical term for this is "hyperalgesia," which is a fancy medical term meaning an increased painful response—a super-sensitivity—to a stimulus that is already usually painful. Or to put it more graphically, if the normal response would be "ow," thanks to hyperalgesia, it is now "oooowwwwwwwwcchhh!!!"

Virtually everyone has experienced hyperalgesia. Imagine the slight pain that one feels from scratching a pin across the skin. Now, imagine the pain that scratching a pin across sunburned skin would cause. In both cases, the stimulus is the same. However, the pain resulting from those two stimuli is quite different. In the case of sunburned skin, the pain fibers respond far more vigorously. Sunburn, of course, is not the only type of condition that can lead to hyperalgesia. Almost all injuries do so. This is, in fact, what makes a sore muscle sore.

By now you may be thinking, "That is all very interesting, and could be quite useful if I am ever on a quiz show. But how does that help me control my pain?" Well, it gives you information about one means of reducing pain. When the amount of prostaglandin present around the pain nerve fiber is decreased, hyperalgesia (super-sensitivity to painful stimulus) is reduced. This results in diminished pain.

The question, then, is: "How can prostaglandin be decreased?"

Back to Medicaleze for a minute. Prostaglandin is actually created at sites of injury through a complex chemical process. One of the important steps of that process involves an enzyme named cyclo-oxygenase (pronounced sigh-clo-ox-ee-jen-ace). Enzymes are the marvelous conversion devices in the body that, step by step, assemble or take apart the chemical constituents of the body. If the activity of cyclo-oxygenase is inhibited, the amount of prostaglandin made at the site of disease or injury is diminished. This, in turn, reduces the hyperalgesia. Thus, reducing the amount of prostaglandin at the site of injury (by reducing the activity of cyclo-oxygenase) will reduce pain. Indeed, this is the type of pain control with which most people are familiar.

The best-known drugs that inhibit the activity of cyclo-oxygenase are nonsteroidal anti-inflammatory drugs or NSAIDS. You probably know NSAIDs by more familiar names, such as aspirin, naproxen, and ibuprofen, or by commercial brand names like Advil®, Aleve®, Motrin®, and other over-the-counter and prescription pain remedies. NSAIDs inhibit the cyclo-oxygenase enzyme so less prostaglandin is produced at the sites of disease or injury. The net result is less pain, as anyone who has taken an NSAID for a tension headache or minor arthritis knows.

Side Effects to Watch for

The next question is, "What's the catch?" Ah, yes. The catch. In medicine, it seems there's *always* a catch. It's known as a side effect.

Upset Stomach

As with most other forms of treatment, NSAIDs do have side effects. That's because cyclo-oxygenase (which is inhibited by NSAIDs) does more than increase the sensitivity of pain nerve fibers. It is also essential for certain other body functions that we do not want to inhibit. For example, cyclo-oxygenase prevents stomach acid from causing ulcers. If we impede the activity of cyclo-oxygenase too much or for too long, we increase the risk that the patient will form stomach ulcers. This, in a nutshell, is why stomach irritation is the most common side effect of NSAIDs.

Overcoming the side effects of beneficial drugs is a constant effort of medicine. Interestingly, we have just discovered that the chemical structure of cyclo-oxygenase at sites of inflammation differs from its structure when found in the stomach and kidney. The two known types of cyclo-oxygenase are called, not surprisingly, cyclo-oxyge-nase type 1 and cyclo-oxygenase type 2, or COX-1 and COX-2 for short. (Ah, those imaginative research scientists!) The easy way to remember which one is which is to remember that we have only one stomach, but may have more than one site of inflammation. Thus, COX-1 is the form found in the *one* stomach a person has. That's the kind we don't want to inhibit when we treat pain. COX-2 is the form found at the many sites of inflammation. We do want to inhibit it to reduce or end pain. Inhibiting the activity of COX-2 reduces the amount of prostaglandin made at the sites of injury and/or in-flammation, thereby reducing hyperalgesia, to the end effect that pain is reduced. This variation in the structure of that important enzyme has allowed the chemists at pharmaceutical companies to develop drugs that inhibit one type of cyclo-oxygenase, but not the other type. By not inhibiting the protective activity of COX-1, these medi-cines still treat pain caused by inflammation, but don't upset delicate stomachs.

Only a small minority of people who take NSAIDs develop ul-cers or kidney trouble as a result of taking their pain medicine. That means that not everybody is better off taking COX-2 antagonists rather than traditional NSAIDs. The people at greatest risk for ulcers are those who are malnourished or chronically ill, or with prior history of ulcers or kidney disease. Patients who take NSAIDs for long periods of time are also, not surprisingly, at greater risk of ulcers. On the other hand, people with low risk of stomach upset can usually con-tinue to take traditional NSAIDs.

So why doesn't everyone just take the medicine that doesn't up-set stomachs? One reason is money. That's another issue that is ever-present when deciding the kinds of medical treatments to pursue or reject. Medicine that only inhibits COX-2 are currently much more expensive than the older NSAIDs, which inhibit both COX-1 and COX-2. In this time of rising medical costs, doctors have a duty to use resources wisely, and thus most prefer to prescribe the more expensive medicine only for patients who are at particularly high risk of complications from NSAID therapy. Moreover, insurance companies, particularly health maintenance organizations (HMOs) or other managed care programs, may insist upon it.

Still, there are many people taking traditional NSAIDs today who would be better off with COX-2 pain relievers. If you suffer significant side effects from the normal kind of aspirin or brand name NSAIDs, you may wish to bring this issue up with your doctor. There are two COX-2 pain remedies currently marketed in the United States, Celebrex® (the generic name is celecoxib) and Vioxx® (the generic name is rofecoxib). There will undoubtedly be more such drugs in the future, and it is likely that the supplier competition in this market will drive down the prices in the future.

The other reason that not everyone taking NSAIDs should switch to COX-2 pain relievers is the enormous variability among people in their response to medication. For reasons not completely understood, some patients experience greater pain relief from traditional NSAIDs than from those only affecting COX-2 enzymes. In fact, even within the category of NSAIDs, there are patients who get relief or side effects from some remedies but not others. It's nearly impossible to predict which patient will have the best response to which drug. Therefore, doctors must sometimes resort to a series of therapeutic trials of different drugs to relieve the patient's pain. "Therapeutic trials"— that's doctor talk for "trial and error."

Toxicity

Toxicity is another potential problem with these drugs. Toxicity means that the compound in question has the potential to damage an organ. With regard to NSAIDs, kidneys are susceptible to harm from the toxic effect of these drugs. At most risk are patients with kidney disease. Also, patients with diabetes, high blood pressure, or who are taking other medications that also have the potential to harm kidneys, should work carefully with their doctors to monitor their kidney functions. That holds true for older patients as well, since kidney function normally declines with age. Thus, "old age" itself, may be looked upon as a condition potentially associated with kidney damage. NSAIDs also have the potential to cause toxic damage to the liver.

This being so, people who regularly take these drugs should be on the alert. For example, elderly people who may take aspirin daily for arthritis or other relatively minor aches and pains associated with growing old, should be careful, as should heart patients who may have been prescribed aspirin for its blood-thinning qualities as a way to avoid a heart attack. If your doctor has mentioned that toxicity is a problem for you, be sure to work closely with your medical team to ensure that your pain control doesn't cause ongoing damage to your kidneys, liver or other organs. In this regard, do not make the mistake of confusing bladder function with kidney function. Just because you are able to urinate without difficulty does not mean that your kidneys are equally robust. That is why regular blood tests of your kidney and liver function may be important if you are taking NSAIDs for extended periods. Thus, don't become complacent about side effects just because the drug you take is as seemingly safe as aspirin.

 ### _From the Doctor's Journal:_

A friend of mine is a pain specialist in another state. We ran into each other at a symposium where we were both lecturing. Over a few beers, and late into the night, we shared "war stories" about our successes—and our failures.

He told me about one of the most frustrating cases he had encountered. The patient was his father-in-law. He described him as a crusty but lovable old timer, not given to frivolous complaints. When he developed gout, an extremely painful arthritis affecting his big toe, he sought my friend's advice.

Now the management of gout is fairly straightforward. The disease results from crystals of uric acid forming in the joint fluid between bones. One part of the treatment, therefore, is preventative: reduce the amount of uric acid in the blood, and there will be a lower likelihood of it precipitating in the joint. But that is only half the battle. There's a reason why the disease's nickname is "gouch." To reduce the terrible pain in the foot, anti-inflammatory drugs or, rarely, even stronger analgesics are needed.

My friend's approach to the problem was the same one I would have selected. He first tried the usually prescribed remedies for his father-in-law. No luck. Either they didn't work, or they caused intolerable side effects. He tried the second-line agents, and then the third-line ones. Still no luck. At that point, the patient thanked his son-in-law for his efforts, and dropped out of his care.

I could sympathize with my buddy. Most doctors don't like treating their family members. But when one has a medical problem within the doctor's specialty, it's hard to resist or refuse to do so. Besides, in-laws seem to be borderline cases: they're close enough to be called family, but not so close that the doctor loses perspective entirely in caring for them. And how does one tell his wife that her fancy specialist husband can't help her father?

The conclusion of the story drives home the point about individual response to therapy. A few weeks after leaving my friend's care, his father-in-law announced to him that his foot was all better. "Marvelous!" exclaimed my friend, "How did you accomplish that?" Perhaps another specialist, he thought, was consulted and came up with an innovative new therapy for the father-in-law's gout.

"The girl at the checkout counter in the drug store recommended I try Aleve®," he said. "It worked like a charm."
Aleve® is a trade name for naproxen, one of the older NSAIDs.
It is sold over the counter for a few pennies a pill. By chance,
that was not among the medicines that my friend had tried in
treating his father-in-law.

One of the best pain medicine specialists in America
had been "out-doctored" by a high school girl working as a
clerk in a drug store. I'd call it a pity, but for two facts. First,
his father-in-law felt better. Second, anything that helps keep a
doctor humble cannot be a complete waste.

NSAIDs might be called medicine's first line of defense
against pain. They effectively treat mild to moderate pain, but are
usually not strong enough to provide significant relief for severe
pain. They are convenient, readily available in the familiar over-
the-counter forms as well as in stronger, prescription-strength
formulas.

A major deficiency concerning NSAIDs has little to do with
the activity of the drugs themselves, although, as mentioned earlier, side effects should be kept firmly in mind and monitored as
your doctor recommends. The biggest problem is that, too often,
they are prescribed to treat pain for which they are ineffective.
That is, doctors may stop with NSAIDs when prescribing to alleviate pain, and simply shrug their shoulders when their patients
receive inadequate relief. Such self-limitation is unacceptable, and
leads to much suffering. So, if these drugs work for you and the
side effects are appropriately limited, that's great. But if you don't

get the relief you need, it does not mean you are doomed to suffer. There are other, more powerful drugs that have the potential to erase even the most severe forms of pain as well as other pain relief treatments that offer great hope for people in even the most pronounced agony. These will be discussed in the next chapters.

CHAPTER 4

———————■———————

Morphine:
Miracle Drug Against Pain

"Among the remedies which it has pleased Almighty God to give man to relieve his suffering, none is so universal and so efficacious as opium."

Sydenham, 1680

Uncontrollable pain. The very notion is enough to cause fear and trembling. Most people wouldn't wish unstoppable agony on their worst enemies. Indeed, if there were such a thing as a fate worse than death, for most people it would be dying in uncontrollable, unremitting, agonizing pain.

The fear of uncontrollable pain is not irrational. Before the advent of modern medicine, people suffered terribly from a myriad of painful conditions, and doctors had precious little to offer to alleviate the suffering. But the last century was a time of astonishing medical advances, among them being the vast improvement in our ability to eliminate or substantially alleviate pain. Albert Schweitzer once remarked that pain is a more terrible lord of mankind than death itself. At long last, we can topple that terrible lord from his pedestal.

Despite these wonderful medical breakthroughs, people still worry terribly about suffering uncontrollable pain. Are these fears groundless? Unfortunately, no. To say factually that medical science knows how to eliminate or substantially alleviate pain is not the same thing as saying that virtually all pain is being successfully eliminated or substantially alleviated. Sadly, contemporary medicine often does a terrible job of treating serious pain. As a consequence, far too many people have helplessly watched loved ones writhe in pain, or have suffered such misery themselves.

The studies are numerous and unequivocal about the failure of modern medicine to perform up to its capability. For example, Charles Cleeland and co-workers at the University of Wisconsin reported on a survey of cancer pain control in the *New England Journal of Medicine* in 1994. They found that 42 percent of the patients were receiving inadequate pain relief. The serious pain of elderly people in nursing homes is also often neglected. A study by R. Bernabei and co-researchers, published in 1998 in the *Journal of the American Medical Association*, looked at the pain management of elderly cancer patients admitted to a nursing home. A full 29 percent of these dying patients reported daily pain. This is an American disgrace!

Most scandalous of all is that much of the cause of this medical underperformance is the prejudice and ignorance among both doctors and patients about the most effective family of pain-controlling medications available today, leading to their massive underuse and, hence, the inadequate treatment of serious pain. Drugs in this category are known as "opioids"—the most famous of which is morphine.

Opioid is the modern name for that class of drugs that used to be called narcotics. A new name was needed, because the word "narcotic" became associated with "getting high," drug addiction, and street crime. In the context of pain treatment, such associations are false and misleading.

Opioids are drugs that mimic the action of certain chemicals found normally in the human brain and spinal cord that work naturally to inhibit pain. The wonder is not that the human nervous system makes chemicals that work like morphine. As described earlier, the body manufactures an array of chemicals that inhibit or reduce the sensation of pain. The real miracle—one on which we frequently reflect and from which we take great comfort—is that the poppy plant manufactures similar drugs that mimic the effect of the natural human "pain-relief hormone." Properly used, these plant extracts and their synthetic relatives can eliminate some of the worst pain that humans suffer.

Opioids work similarly to their naturally occurring counterparts in the human body. As mentioned earlier, when soldiers seriously injured in battle say that they felt no pain, only the sense of a minor wound, they are not exaggerating. In these cases, the pain stimulus is present, but the spinal cord blocks the transmission of pain signals from the site of injury to the brain. Natural morphine-like chemicals, which are secreted in the spinal cord and brain, cause the blocking of the pain signal. Simply put, morphine and other opioid drugs kill pain by mimicking this natural function.

Debunking the Myths about Morphine

Despite their wondrous properties, morphine and other opioids are medicine's most underutilized pain treatment. Part of this problem is caused by the vast network of federal and state laws and regulations that govern the use of opioids, known in government parlance as "controlled substances." Many doctors report that fear of prosecution creates a "chilling effect," discouraging aggressive and effective pain control in too many instances. Others object to the bureaucratic burdens placed on doctors willing to prescribe opioids for pain. For example, some states require that prescriptions for narcotics be filled out in triplicate, with the state government receiving a copy of each prescription. These triplicate prescription forms seldom serve any useful regulatory function. Yet, in states where it is required, the triplicate form's chilling effect persists, creating fear among doctors that there will be a knock on the door by regulatory authorities. Other states require doctors to pay several hundred dollars extra per year to be able to prescribe opioids for their patients.

Another problem, as unbelievable as it sounds, is that most doctors do not receive adequate training in medical school or residency on the proper use of these drugs to control pain. Consequently, lacking even the knowledge to know what they don't know, many doctors fail to turn to these drugs when their patients' pain requires it. Others are afraid to engage in proper pain treatment out of a misguided worry that they will hurt the patient more than help them with these drugs.

These and other circumstances that hinder the legitimate use of morphine and similar drugs cry out for reform. That is not to say that the government should not control and regulate the use of opioids. It should. But there needs to be a broader recognition, by both doctors and patients, of the relative safety and effectiveness of opioids. And organized medicine must commit itself to ensuring that no doctor remains unaware of the benefits of opioids or untrained in their proper use.

Advocating for needed legal reform and promoting specific changes in medical school curricula are beyond the scope of this book. However, dispelling baseless fears and exposing false conceptions about opioids are definitely in order and will take up the balance of this chapter.

A primary reason for the underuse of opioids is that certain myths hamper doctors from prescribing them aggressively. Similarly, and tragically, many patients are more afraid of morphine and other opioids than they are of their own terrible pain. Making matters worse, nurses and other support staff may worry that proper dosing of morphine in hospitals is improper, leading them to resist cooperating with proper medical protocols. The consequence: pain exercises power over people instead of people exercising power over pain.

The time has come to get rid of fear and ignorance about morphine and other opioids. We must learn the truth about opioids as proper medicine in controlling pain. We must ensure that doctors, patients, government regulators, and medical staffs embrace these miracle drugs of nature and allow them to exercise their proper role in relieving cruel human suffering.

 ## From the Doctor's Journal:

"The truth will set you free." When I first started to practice pain medicine at my hospital, my aggressive use of opioids made many nurses uncomfortable. Unsure about whether the seemingly high doses of morphine I was prescribing were safe for them to administer, some worried that my intention was other than therapeutic, that I intended these high doses of morphine to kill, rather than treat, my cancer patients.

God forbid!

That led to some controversy, not only with nurses but also with pharmacists whom the nurses called to report their concerns. I knew that I had an education project at hand, so I patiently explained to them my benign therapeutic intent, and how these doses would achieve it.

It did not take long, fortunately, for the nurses and pharmacists to understand that my opioid-intensive approach to pain control worked! The patients didn't stop breathing; they stopped moaning! They became more mobile and interactive. The nurses and pharmacists, as dedicated health care professionals, shared in the joy of seeing our patients achieve a comfort they had not known for too long, and which many had thought they would never know again.

I don't get so many worried phone calls from nurses now. Now the nurses wonder why other doctors don't prescribe higher doses of opioid analgesics. So do I.

Truth 1: Morphine Use Is Safe

It is commonly believed that aggressive use of morphine and other opioid drugs carries a high risk of killing patients. The myth that morphine and other such drugs are unsafe is caused by failing to distinguish opioid effects in different groups of people. It is true that, when people who do not have pain are given narcotics, the drugs carry the risk of suppressing the respiratory drive, making it so people do not breathe. Even patients who have pain but who are just beginning opioid therapy (called "opioid-naïve" patients by doctors) must be dosed carefully to prevent this effect. Fortunately, the body becomes used to these drugs fairly quickly, usually in a matter of a few days or weeks. After that, the sedating effect of the opioid subsides, as does its potential to suppress respiration. Thus, opioid doses may usually be raised safely in the patient who has some prior or ongoing exposure to the drug.

Too many people, when they think of morphine use, envision a doctor holding a syringe coming to the patient's bedside to sadly inform him that the shot can relieve his pain, but only by "knocking him out" and probably killing him. That is certainly the picture presented in popular television programs. Rubbish! Absolute rubbish!

The danger attributed to opioids has been wildly exaggerated in the popular consciousness. In fact, deaths caused by the proper medical use of opioids, even in opioid-naïve patients, are strikingly rare. Therefore, rather than worrying unduly about morphine hastening death, the greater danger to human welfare is allowing this myth about opioids to result in undertreated pain. Properly prescribed, morphine and other opioids are more likely to extend life than shorten it, because of the terrible physical and emotional toll that pain exacts on the body. Thus, it is far more compassionate and humane—in other words, it is simply good medical care—to treat pain vigorously, rather than to allow people to writhe in potentially deadly agony.

Truth 2: Morphine Used to Treat Pain Does Not Cause Drug Addiction

Some physicians still refuse to prescribe opioids, and some patients refuse to take them, because they fear addiction. It is true, of course, that pain-controlling medicines can be, and sometimes are, abused. For example, when these drugs are taken in order to induce a state of intoxication rather than to treat pain, they may be addicting. But that societal problem should not deter the proper medical use of these medicines, especially since they *virtually never cause addiction when taken to treat chronic pain.*

Addiction is a psychological as well as a biological disorder. The addict seeks drugs for their mood-altering effect, and will continue to use drugs for this purpose regardless of the deleterious impact on his health, social position, societal function, marriage, etc. A three-word summary of the complex phenomenon of addiction is "use despite harm." Although some addicts go to doctors to get drugs, pain patients who take opioids under a physician's direction do not become addicts as a result. Pain medication properly prescribed does not cause intoxication. It does not cause people to get "high." What it does do is eliminate pain, thereby allowing people to go about their lives unhindered.

The Difference Between Addiction and Dependence

In considering the issue of addiction, we must distinguish addiction from drug dependence. An addicted person takes the drug for its psychological effect. The compulsion to obtain a "fix" may be so strong that addicts will commit crimes to obtain the means to feed their habits. Addiction is characterized by a persistent pattern of dysfunctional drug use. It may involve adverse consequences of drug use, loss of control over the use of the drug, as well as preoccupation with obtaining the drug.

Drug dependence, sometimes called physical dependency, is a distinct phenomenon. Dependence on an opioid is a physiologic state in which abrupt cessation of the opioid results in a withdrawal syndrome. Physical dependency on opioids is an expected occurrence in all individuals who continuously use them in significant doses, whether the drug is used for therapeutic or for non-therapeutic purposes. It does not, in and of itself, imply addiction.

Many drugs cause physical dependency. For example, people who drink coffee in the morning may develop a headache if they don't have their morning cup. That's because they are dependent on caffeine. Withdrawal symptoms occur if the drug is stopped abruptly—that is what being dependent on a drug means. Non-addicted, drug dependent people don't mug old ladies to get their drug, they don't prostitute themselves, and they don't steal from their families because they are desperate for a fix. Patients who are opioid-dependent are not opioid addicts. If and when the time comes to go off the drug, it does not require membership in a 12-step program.

It should be obvious that addiction and dependence can exist independently or together. Some addicts are physically dependent; others are not. Some people who are physically dependent are addicted; others are not. Many people become dependent on opioids, just as many others become dependent on some blood pressure medications, or on steroids used to treat severe arthritis. But we have never seen a non-addicted person become addicted to opioids as a result of using them to treat pain.

The Problem of Pseudo-Addiction

There is a phenomenon that resembles addiction, but must be distinguished from it. That is pseudo-addiction. The pseudo-addict is the person whose drug-seeking behavior is driven by poor pain control. The patient is not seeking to get high, just to obtain relief of pain. Many doctors mistake pseudo-addicts for addicts, and, instead of prescribing adequate doses of opioid pain medicine, prescribe completely inadequate doses of often inadequate drugs—leaving the patient desperate for more drugs to get out of pain.

While true iatrogenic (doctor-caused) addiction is rare, iatrogenic pseudo-addiction is relatively common. Demanding better pain relief is interpreted by the doctors as being a sign of addiction, and, consequently, the patient is prescribed less medicine, or less effective medicine, than what is required to effectively treat the patient's pain. That, in turn, creates a vicious cycle. Improperly treated, the patient remains in pain. Because of pain, the patient requests more pain-relieving medicine. The doctor, fearing the patient is becoming addicted, refuses to adequately prescribe the necessary medication. Then, if the desperate patient, fed up with the inadequate care received from the first doctor, goes to a second or a third doctor, he or she is accused of "doctor-shopping for drugs." This is misinterpreted as further evidence of drug addiction, leading to a downward spiral, including desperation and sometimes suicide.

Pseudo-addiction is a common problem that requires a compassionate solution. The medical and legal systems must learn to distinguish better between appropriate use of opioids for pain relief and improper drug abuse. Until we do, too many people will continue to suffer pain in the name of preventing their addiction.

From the Doctor's Journal:

Some of the most heart-wrenching cases I see are those of pseudo-addiction, because, by definition, it involves a patient who has been misdiagnosed and mistreated. I remember a young woman—let's call her Sally—who suffered from persistent pain on one side of her face. I met her when she was hospitalized because of a crisis in that pain. In many ways she reminded me of my wife. She was the same age, and, like my wife, a woman who found fulfillment in the busy life of being a homemaker and mother of young children. Then disaster struck. Unbeknownst to her, she had an arteriovenous malformation in the brain. That is a cluster of abnormal fragile blood vessels. In Sally's case, the blood vessels burst, leading to emergency neurosurgery and mild, but persistent, weakness on one side. More importantly, the illness led to persistent pain in the face. This is because the blood vessels that burst and the site of the operation had been near the nerve that transmits pain information from the face to the rest of the brain.

Her primary care physician had been in charge of her treatment. He was well meaning, but no specialist in the field. He prescribed Vicodin®, a short-acting opioid in combination with acetaminophen. This was far from ideal, but gave the patient enough relief that she could carry on her daily activities. Perhaps he expected the pain to go away, to be "cured," rather than to be a chronic illness requiring chronic management. In any case, he became uncomfortable when week after week, and month after month, Sally not only needed Vicodin® to control her pain, but she asked for increasing amounts of the drug. She was set up to be a pseudo-addict: she had an obscure pain syndrome, treated with short-acting opioids in inadequate doses.

Sally's primary care doctor referred her to a high-power specialty center a few hours away. There she was admitted to the drug abuse unit! She was informed that she was a drug addict, that the way to recovery was not to focus on the pain, but on the "real issues" that had led to her drug abuse. The opioids were stopped abruptly.

47

Sally believed that she was a full-fledged addict. And why not? All the specialists in the drug abuse unit told her she was addicted, all the nurses reinforced the message, and all the other patients there were clearly addicted. Whenever doubts arose in her mind, she remembered that denial was a hallmark of addiction, ironically reinforcing the very diagnosis she questioned.

It was a tough withdrawal. She experienced chills, shakes, sweats, diarrhea, and abdominal cramps. She thought about the Vicodin®, and how it had helped her pain. And she believed that the withdrawal and her mental state meant she had become a drug addict. Added to the facial pain and the wrenching symptoms of opioid withdrawal was a humiliating sense of shame.

I remember that Sally cried when I told her that she wasn't really an addict, that she was a pseudo-addict, and that there are crucial differences between the two. I must admit, I almost cried too. All that suffering, and so much of it doctor-induced.

Sally is now doing well, enjoying good pain control on a long-acting opioid. She still needs occasional reassurance that she is not addicted. But her husband, whose wife has been restored to him, and her children, whose mommy can again be an active part of their lives, need no such reassurance. They can't give the fancy definitions and distinctions between addiction and pseudoaddiction, but they know that if mommy takes her medicine, she's mommy again, not the pitiful woman who just lies in bed moaning.

Truth 3: Increasing Dosage Does Not Harm the Patient

Another concept related to the addiction issue is that of drug tolerance. Tolerance means that increased doses of a medication are needed to achieve the same previous medical effect. For example, a doctor may initially prescribe 20 mg. per day of an opioid for a patient with chronic, non-malignant pain. A week later, the patients will report good pain control, but in a few weeks, the pain relief has worn off. Raising the dose to 40 mg. per day will restore the pain control for another few weeks, but then again the benefit wears off. Another dose elevation at that point will usually restore pain control, and that dose is often the final one needed.

Tolerance is not an endless process. Most patients (other than terminally ill cancer patients) become tolerant to the opioid during the first few months of therapy, but there is usually little increase in the tolerance after that point. Because this tolerance develops in the early days of opioid therapy, often when the doctor and the patient have not yet established a relationship of mutual trust, the need for repeated dose increases is misinterpreted as being due to drug addiction. Or even worse, the doctor may wrongly suspect that the patient is selling the drug on the black market, a criminal activity known as drug diversion. Better medical education should go far to solve this problem.

Patients with advanced cancer may seem to have ongoing needs for dose escalation. In these cases, however, the need for increased dosages is usually not because of tolerance alone. Rather, it's the worsening of their underlying conditions that causes the need for higher doses of pain medicine. In other words, cancer patients at the end of life may need steadily higher doses because the painful stimulus has increased, not just because of opioid tolerance.

From the Doctor's Journal:

The most extreme example of tolerance I have seen involves a young woman with advanced metastatic cancer. Fortunately, she is receiving excellent hospice care. She is a deeply religious woman who wanted to spend her final days at home, with her husband and young children, and with frequent visits by church members. When her cancer pain became difficult to manage, the hospice nurses recommended to her primary care physician that a pain specialist be consulted. To his credit, that physician continued the supportive medical relationship he had long maintained with the patient, and supplemented it by consultation with a pain specialist.

At first, the case seemed simple enough. With progressive cancer, her pain had worsened, and she simply needed higher doses of opioids. Over time, however, the character of the pain changed. In addition to her previous abdominal and back pain, she developed pain in the arm that she said felt like jolts of electricity (neuropathy). I suspected that she had nerve damage of a kind that does not respond well to opioids. (She was too ill to travel to a diagnostic center.) So I added a drug that is beneficial in treating neuropathic pain to her previous pain control regimen. Thus, while the opioids controlled her tissue damage pain, we also controlled her nerve damage pain.

Finally, the patient developed difficulty in swallowing. That put her at risk for both untreated pain and opioid withdrawal. The answer to that challenge was to deliver her pain control through a tiny pump. I inserted a small needle, about the size used by diabetics to inject insulin, under her skin (but not in a vein). Through it was infused a small but steady volume of hydromorphone, a concentrated potent opioid.

50

That did the trick. In fact, with good pain control, she rallied to the point of getting up out of bed and going to church. The pump was carried discretely under her clothes.

Her high dose of hydromorphone reflects several things—the severity of her illness, her tolerance to opioids, and their safety, even in high doses, in patients who are tolerant to them. She is now receiving 100 mg. per hour of subcutaneous hydromorphone. This is approximately equivalent to 36,000 mg. of oral morphine per day. To give you a sense of how high this dose is, consider that it is a thousand times higher than the dose needed by many cancer patients to achieve good pain control.

Is it a high dose? To be sure. Is it too high? Not for this patient. For her it is just right.

Truth 4: Opioid Use Now Will Not Render Later Use Ineffective

The issue of tolerance also comes up in another context. People with progressing diseases such as cancer are often reluctant to treat their pain aggressively because they worry that, when their condition worsens, their pain control will cease to be effective.

Happily, the opposite is true. If pain increases, so can the safe dose of opioid needed to control the pain. One reason, of course, is that even people without pain will become tolerant to the sedating effect of opioids if they receive them over a prolonged period. Another reason is that pain is a powerful stimulant. Opioids, on the other hand, are depressants. If the stimulus of pain is greater, a higher dose of opioid is both needed and tolerated to bring relief. Thus, people with an advancing painful cancer can safely take morphine or other opioids in increasing doses that might otherwise be unsafe for them to take. This interesting interaction means that there is no automatic upper limit to the opioid dose that can be safely provided to the patient in severe pain. This means that even the most painful conditions are capable of effective control.

 ### *From the Doctor's Journal:*

This stimulating effect of pain was brought home to me in a powerful way. I was treating an elderly woman with metastatic breast cancer. Initially, she had fair pain control on oral morphine. But her comfort declined considerably when she broke her hip due to the cancer. She was admitted to the hospital, and was placed on intravenous morphine rather than oral morphine, so that we might more rapidly adjust the dose of the medicine to control the pain. Frankly, we were not satisfied with the results. The drug was causing some side effects, and the pain control, while adequate, was nothing to brag about. Since her pain came mainly from disease in her pelvis and hips, I thought she would do better with morphine given directly into the spinal fluid through a slender catheter inserted in her lower back. That way, the pain blocking effect of the morphine could be delivered where the pain signals were entering the spinal cord, with less drug delivered to her brain.

She had been a little sleepy from the morphine before the spinal therapy, but almost within minutes of receiving the pain relief from the spinal therapy, she became deeply asleep. Fortunately, her respiration remained well within a safe range. The spinal therapy had abruptly stopped the arousing pain signals from reaching her brain. The dose of intravenous morphine being given was now unopposed by pain, and, therefore, was now quite sedating to her. My challenge was to taper the dose of the intravenous morphine rapidly, to allow her to wake up completely, but not so rapidly as to precipitate withdrawal. The spinal therapy had precipitated the sleepiness but was not its cause. The cause was the sudden cessation of pain to oppose the sedating effect of the intravenous morphine. The proof of this is that she became quite alert with tapering of the intravenous dose, with no adjustment of the spinal dose.

■

Truth 5: The Need for Strong Pain Control Does Not Mean Death Is Near

An understandable myth that is sometimes a barrier to the successful management of chronic pain is the fear of prognostic implications. In other words, patients with life-threatening conditions may think, "Gee, if the doctor is prescribing morphine for me, I must really be a goner!" So worried are some patients about the "bad news" meaning of needed pain control, that they will underreport their pain to their doctors. The subconscious rationale is that if the doctor doesn't prescribe it, then "I don't need it," and that means, "I'm going to live longer." In fact, the choice of morphine or other opioid to treat chronic pain has nothing to do, in and of itself, with the prognosis. It has everything to do with the severity of the pain. The two issues should not be confused.

 From the Doctor's Journal:

Just as cancer was once referred to as "the big C," so some clinicians jokingly refer to morphine as "the M word." Hollywood has worked its magic on us all. We've seen too many movies in which the administration of morphine was a handy metaphor for impending death. (Keep in mind that the film writers are even worse educated about pain medicine than most doctors, which is to say very poorly educated.) It is not unusual for me to encounter patients who prefer the oxycodone found in Percocet® to morphine to treat their pain, not because it is a better drug for their particular need, but because the name is less scary. They are surprised to learn that in fact oral oxycodone is about twice the potency of oral morphine.

Truth 6: Morphine Does Not Cause Stupor

Many people are reluctant to take morphine or other opioids because they worry about living their lives in a drug-induced haze or stupor. This is sometimes called the "zombie" myth, because patients are afraid the drug will turn them into a zombie. This fear, like so many others, is misguided. While it is true that patients taking opioids for pain control may feel drowsy during the first few days of therapy, for the vast majority of them that adverse effect diminishes dramatically within a short time. In the minority of cases in which the dose necessary to relieve pain is simply too sedating, the addition of a stimulant drug may make the difference between therapeutic success and failure.

Opioids properly prescribed do not cause stupor. In fact, the opposite is true. People, who have for years—sometimes decades—been in unremitting and merciless pain, can get relief by proper therapy. Their lives will not be distorted or ruined by drug therapy. Rather, it is the pain which has been ruining their lives and distorting their personalities. With proper therapy, be it opioid or other therapy, patients can regain control of their lives. Unfortunately, the English language does not have a word for "the opposite of a zombie." If there were such a word, we would use it now to describe what people can become with proper therapy of their pain.

 ### *From the Doctor's Journal:*

One of the pleasures of my practice is to see the emergence of a personality that has been obscured by pain. I began treating a middle-aged woman for severe arm pain following an injury. Initially, she was whiney, depressed, and focused on her pain. Frankly, she was not very likable then.

At first, the treatment did not go well. The initial medications were either ineffective or caused unacceptable side effects. I became discouraged, and felt the need in my own heart for a "boost" to keep me going in the case. I asked the patient's husband to tell me what she had been like before the injury. I was amazed to hear the description, for it was the opposite of the impression I had formed of the same woman. He described her as fun loving, light-hearted, with an impish sense of humor.

That was the clue I needed. I decided to go on a treasure hunt. Like an archaeologist sifting through mud in order to find a buried treasure, I continued to search for the light-hearted woman within the suffering person I saw before me.

Gradually she emerged. As her pain subsided, her functional status improved. She came into my office smiling instead of crying. She brought in photos of her beloved dogs and father (yes, it was in that order). She began to tell jokes. It was not simply that her husband found it a pleasure to be with her again. More importantly, she found it a pleasure to be with herself again.

The myths about opioids lead to scandalous levels of undertreated pain, causing untold human misery. Too many people—physicians and patients alike—allow these myths to prevent aggressive and proper medical care of patients in terrible pain. The time has come to eliminate this ignorance and superstition and bring relief to millions of suffering people.

Understanding Opioid Side Effects

Opioids are medicine, and any medicine has the potential for side effects. The good news is that these side effects, once recognized, can be managed (reduced or eliminated), just like the side effects of other classes of drugs. With proper management, side effects do not preclude successful management of serious pain.

Sedation

One side effect of concern is sedation. Most patients who are taking opioids for the first time, or who are significantly increasing the dose in the face of chronic use, will experience temporary drowsiness. This is usually mild, and, as mentioned earlier in this chapter, subsides after a few days. Part of the drowsiness probably comes from the fact that people in chronic pain do not sleep well. They may be likened to college students who have stayed up studying all night before a big examination. If you put these students in a dark room with a soft bed, they are soon fast asleep. Similarly, when people in chronic pain finally get some relief from suffering, they can get caught up on some lost and badly needed sleep. This is not the only factor causing sleepiness when opioid therapy is started, but it is one of them.

In occasional cases, patients with chronic pain continue to have intolerable sedation as a side effect of opioids at the dose they need to control their pain. *That does not mean that the patient's only choice is to be sleepy and out of pain, or wakeful and in pain.* In these circumstances, it is reasonable for the doctor to *prescribe a drug to maintain wakefulness and continue the opioid therapy.* While it seems against the usual rules of medicine to prescribe a drug simply to relieve the side effects of another drug (rather than replacing the original, offending drug), the reason this is done is that, for many people, there simply is no other class of drug that provides the necessary level of pain relief.

Nausea

Another possible side effect of opioids is nausea. Fortunately, this is not a problem for most patients. For those who do develop upset stomachs, the problem is usually mild and short-term. Most patients need no medical intervention at all, except for counseling, to put up with the side effect for the few days it will be present. Others need to take a mild anti-nausea medicine for a few days. In rare cases, the nausea does not improve after a few days, and becomes a limiting factor in the treatment of the patient. In these cases, for reasons not well understood (in fact, not understood at all), the patient may do well on a different opioid. For example, there are patients who develop intractable nausea on morphine, but who do fine on oxycodone. While this is rare, some patients, who cannot tolerate the first, second, or even the third opioid prescribed, achieve both significant pain relief and freedom from nausea with the fourth opioid drug prescribed. *The key point in this, as in other aspects of pain medicine, is not to give up.* If the first prescribed drug causes unacceptable side effects that do not end and cannot be alleviated, ask your doctor to try a different drug.

Constipation

Constipation is the most common side effect of morphine and other opioid medicines. Unlike the other side effects we have addressed, constipation does *not* get better with time. However, constipation caused by opioids is, itself, eminently treatable with laxatives and diet control.

Unless the patient already has chronic diarrhea, or is likely to require only low doses of opioids, *laxatives should be started at the same time as the opioid*. Senna compounds or lactulose are commonly prescribed to treat opioid induced constipation. The important thing is not which drug is taken to prevent constipation, but that a laxative be taken, and taken regularly. Most patients who need laxatives will continue to need them throughout the course of their opioid treatment.

Jerking Movements

"Myoclonic jerks" are another potential side effect. (No, we are not referring to your brothers-in-law.) This is the name given to sudden jerking movements of the arm or leg that may occur when people take high doses of morphine. Healthy people sometimes experience myoclonic jerks, also, as they fall asleep. They may actually awaken a person, or his spouse, and lead to interesting discussions that start with the angry demand, "Why the heck did you kick me?"

When the myoclonic jerks are due to high dose morphine, there are several ways to handle that problem. First, the patient may be reassured that the myoclonic jerks are not seizures, and do not herald seizures. Second, if the twitches do not bother the patient, they really don't need to be treated. If the problem does cause concern, however, it can be eliminated or vastly reduced with the use of another drug, clonazepam. Your doctor may add this prescription safely to the regimen of pain control, allowing pain to be controlled without your experiencing significant myoclonic jerks. Finally, if that isn't effective, your doctor can prescribe an equally effective opioid in place of morphine, since the myoclonic jerks are most commonly seen with high dose morphine, and seldom seen with high doses of other opioids.

Low Testosterone

Opioids commonly have another side effect that remains virtually unmentioned in the literature pain physicians read. That side effect is low blood levels of testosterone in men who take moderate to high doses of opioids. The reason is that the opioid diminishes the amount of a controlling hormone secreted by the pituitary, a tiny but important gland located at the base of the brain. This hormone, called LH (for luteinizing hormone), directs the testicles to make testosterone. The symptoms of a low testosterone level may include lack of energy, hot flashes, sweating spells, diminished interest in sex, and impotence. The diagnosis is easy. A simple blood test will reveal whether the patient's testosterone level is normal. The treatment is just as easy. The missing hormone may be administered by periodic injections in the buttock, or by daily application of a patch or gel. Even if patients do not experience these symptoms, it is probably worth checking for low testosterone levels in patients who are not terminally ill. Low testosterone levels are associated with an increased risk of osteoporosis (thinning of the bones). That is now an avoidable complication of opioid therapy.

Death

Can opioids be fatal? Very rarely, yes. But to put the matter in perspective, so can penicillin or over-the-counter medications. The key to safe use of opioids is to use them as prescribed in proper dose. As a patient gets used to opioids, the safety of their use and the ability to increase the dose, if needed, rises considerably. Even at the end of life, when the respiratory drive is diminished by impending death, it is safe to continue opioid therapy if it is needed to control terminal symptoms. In fact, there is often a need for a dramatic dose escalation in the last few days of life. Since the patient is dying, and the dying process itself leads to a greater need for opioids, it is easy to mistake the drug use, instead of the patient's underlying illness or injury, as being the cause of death.

From the Doctor's Journal:

I admitted an elderly female patient with advanced breast cancer from a nursing home to the hospital because of uncontrolled shortness of breath. I thought that she had a day or two to live. I planned to use morphine to treat her terminal symptoms, since the drug diminishes the suffering of shortness of breath, too. I carefully explained to the patient's family (she was not well enough to participate in the conversation) that my prescribing morphine was intended to control symptoms, not to hasten her death, but that it was likely she would die soon. I didn't want them to mistake the morphine as the cause of her death, rather than a palliation of her terminal symptoms.

She had been on moderate doses of oral morphine before her admission to the hospital. She was no longer able to swallow, so I administered the drug intravenously in a somewhat higher equivalent dose.

To my delight and surprise, she did not die that day. Rather, her respirations became more comfortable (and, incidentally, more efficient), and she regained the ability to communicate with her family. Within a few days she was well enough to leave the hospital.

Pain Control Without a Ceiling

A wonderful and unique characteristic of opioids is that they have no "ceiling effect." The same cannot be said for other pain-controlling drugs. For them, the benefit increases as the dose is raised—but only up to a point. Beyond that, the law of diminishing returns kicks in, and the drug has no greater benefit, only increased side effects.

Aspirin is a perfect example of the ceiling effect. As described in Chapter 3, aspirin is a useful drug in the treatment of mild to moderate inflammatory pain. For most people, two aspirin work significantly better than one to control pain, with little additional side effects. Three work a little better than two, but at the price of significantly more toxicity. At that point, aspirin's effectiveness hits a wall. Four or five aspirin work no better than two or three at controlling pain, but have the potential to create far more significant side effects. That is why we say that there is a "ceiling" on the dosage of aspirin. Pushing the dose through that ceiling does not yield any additional benefit and can only result in increased risk of harm. Thus, if two aspirin are not enough to control the pain, five will not be either.

Opioids, in contrast, have no ceiling effect. For most people, the pain-controlling effect increases with increasing the dose, virtually without limit. Then why can't opioids, at one dose or another, completely control everyone's pain? Although there is no uniform ceiling beyond which therapeutic benefit is lost, for most people there is a threshold beyond which side effects do emerge and become problematic. Happily, most pain can be controlled before this point is reached, even pain that is increasing with time and thus requiring higher doses of opioids. For this reason, morphine and other opioids can be increased seemingly without limit to match escalating pain. The limit of the dose in opioids, unlike that of most other drugs, is not a ceiling of lost efficacy, but a variable limit of side effects. *This is why management of opioid side effects is such a key part of proper opioid therapy.* Proper management of side effects increases the amount of opioid the patient can tolerate, thus permitting greater levels of palliation. The increment in dosage allowed by the control of side effects may make the difference between success and failure in pain management.

The lack of ceiling effect also explains the enormous variation in doses that different patients need to achieve satisfactory pain control. Many patients can have good pain control on 60 mg. per day of oral morphine or its equivalent in other opioids. But for some patients, their pain requires dosages literally a hundred times greater than that. Because there is no ceiling effect, opioids can be prescribed at these high doses, particularly when side effects are controlled. In no other class of drug does one see this huge variation in dosing to achieve maximal benefit, which is one reason why opioids are so successful in treating even the most intractable pain.

Since too many doctors have not been adequately trained in controlling pain, they are uninformed, or worse, misinformed, about the lack of ceiling effect. They may express alarm at hearing how high an opioid dose a patient needs for pain control. Even those, who have read some of the modern medical literature about opioid therapy and intellectually understand the lack of ceiling effect and variable opioid dosing, are astounded when they meet and converse with patients taking "huge" doses of morphine. ("Huge" is in quotation marks because, for these patients, the dose is not at all huge; it is just right.) Doctors need to get through the emotional shock of seeing patients who are comfortably taking, and benefiting from, doses of opioids that would be lethal in patients with lower dose requirements or who have not developed tolerance to the drug.

Dosing of opioids is not like paint-by-the-numbers or playing musical scales. Rather, like freehand art or jazz, each attempt at palliation will be different. Each requires individualized skill and precision on the part of the doctor to match the individual needs of the patient. What the doctor and patient are looking for is the dose that best relieves the pain with the least side effects. Moreover, pain control is a dynamic enterprise. From time to time, often for reasons we don't know, the amount of pain a person has will increase or decrease. Like a dancer reacting to a shift in the music, the doctor, too, should respond by increasing or decreasing the dose of opioid to ensure that pain control remains balanced properly to maximize patient benefit and minimize risk.

Morphine and other opioids are not the appropriate treatment for every form of serious pain. However, they are wonderful enhancers of life for millions of people who would otherwise be in agonizing pain. Furthermore, people in serious pain need to be able to discuss the use of opioids with their doctors without fear or shame. We will come back to morphine and other opioids when we discuss the control of pain caused by specific diseases and injuries.

CHAPTER 5

Power over Chronic Pain

Many of the readers of this book are victims of significant discrimination. We are talking about a silent but insidious discrimination, one that is not based on ill will, bigotry, or prejudice. The discrimination is not organized, nor do hate groups dedicate themselves to keeping this minority group down. In fact, most of those who discriminate are not even aware that they are doing so.

From the Doctor's Journal:

I remember one patient who was the victim of two of the few bigotries that can be displayed in otherwise polite company. She was in chronic pain, and she was obese.

"Moonbeam" was in her thirties, and came to see me from a neighboring state. She had terrible knee pain. The cause was obvious. Those knees were never intended to bear over three hundred pounds of weight, and the wear and tear of the years led to disabling pain that impaired her walking. It became, quite literally, a vicious circle: the less she walked, the heavier she got, and the heavier she got, the less she walked. By the time she came to me, she used a wheelchair when going any considerable distance.

The advice of her doctors—"just lose some weight"— was no more compassionate than it was practical. The cure rate for obesity is less than that for cancer.

I treated Moonbeam with sustained-release oxycodone, an opioid pain reliever. Now, I am used to my patients improving dramatically, but she achieved the level of "no pain at all." When she told me she had zero pain, I quizzed her sharply, "Surely it must hurt a little?" I asked. "Nope, doc, not at all," she replied. "Just a smidge?" I suggested. "Unh-unh. None."

No longer held back by knee pain, Moonbeam began to walk…and walk…and walk. She went hiking and camping in forests near her home. And the more she walked, the less she weighed. With each change in dress size—she began wearing dresses again, instead of baggy overalls to hide her shape—she grinned from ear to ear.

After several years of unemployment due to chronic pain, she is now back in the work force, putting in about thirty hours per week. She tells me that she has saved her old "fat photos," and that her goal is to become an "after" in a Jenny Craig Program® advertisement.

We won't tell, will we?

Lack of malice does not make discrimination any less painful. The prejudice about which we write—that imposed against those who suffer from chronic pain—causes the afflicted to lose their jobs, their friends, and sometimes their marriages. Ask chronic pain sufferers how often their pain has been dismissed as imaginary, or discounted as hypochondria. Ask them how their woe has been dismissed by doctors, and disbelieved by employers as an excuse for laziness or shirking of duties. Inquire about how many times the pain sufferer has snapped at a spouse or child, not because of anger, but just because it hurt so damn bad, and the pain would not go away! Ask about how many husbands or wives of the afflicted fail to understand that it is not the end of love or loss of physical attraction, but rather the enduring, unending pain that causes shortness of temper or a lack of romantic drive.

 ### From the Doctor's Journal:

Before I became a pain medicine specialist, I limited my practice to treating cancer and blood diseases. One of the things about treating chronic pain, I noticed, is its similarity to cancer. No, the diseases are not identical, far from it. But their overall impact often is. In both diseases, the clinician must recognize that the family as a whole, not just the identified patient, is suffering. The disease affects a wide circle of people, and helping the one often indirectly helps the many.

"Jo" had once been a vivacious mother and housewife, but, when I met her, she had barely been out of the house in seven years. After an accident, doctors had been unable to save her leg, despite valiant efforts and several operations. It had to be amputated above the knee. She learned to walk with a prosthesis, but often would take it off when her chronic leg pain was particularly bad.

She described the pain as having two components. She had a constant, dull, achy pain in the stump as well as jolts of pain that raced from the stump down to her foot, a part of her body that was no longer there. This is called phantom limb pain, and Jo's was so awful that it made her cry out. She could recall to the minute when a series of jolts started, or when, mercifully, they stopped. The pain, quite literally, made her miserable, and it adversely impacted every close relationship she had.

Just as her pain had two components, it needed to be treated with more than one pain reliever. I treated her with a combination of anti-epileptic medicine and an opioid. The treatment was very successful, and I was subsequently blessed to witness what I called the "flowering of Jo."

Even good news can be a shock and require an adjustment. At first Jo didn't know what to do with herself and her newfound pain relief. She had been fond of gourmet cooking so, early in her recovery, she invited her family over for her once-famous omelets. Not too long after that, she took her grandson on a long-promised but never really expected trip to Niagara Falls.

The full extent of her recovery and her previous disability, however, did not become apparent until several months later, when she saw me on a routine follow-up visit. She was doing quite well by that time, and I had reduced the frequency of her office visits. Jo was a woman who spoke in plain language, so I must paraphrase her conversation, since this is a book intended for a family audience. She announced to me that she had made love with her husband the evening before our visit. "That's nice," I replied, not quite grasping the import of what she had just told me. "No, you don't understand, Doc," she declared. "I always used to hurt too much to even think about sex. Doc, we haven't done it in seven years!"

And then she smiled brightly and, quite charmingly, blushed.

■

Chronic Pain Is as Chronic Pain Does

Anyone who suffers from chronic pain does not need us to explain what it is. They experience it every day as constant, unwanted agony. Still, we are, respectively, a doctor and a lawyer, and for us not to define our terms would bring on cases of itchy hives. More importantly, by realizing that chronic pain is a definable term, readers will better understand that the condition is a diagnosable medical malady, for which there are well-defined treatment protocols.

Medical textbooks take various approaches to define chronic pain. Some definitions require that the pain last for a specified period of time. Others take the approach that the failure of a certain number of pain treatments is the best indication that the patient's pain is chronic. But the approach that works best for our purposes is to define chronic pain as *pain that is not going to get better by itself*, that is, pain that has become a permanent aspect of the patient's life.

Take, for example, a patient who has had unremitting low back pain ever since falling on an ice-covered sidewalk ten years previously. The man has had surgery and traction, and has even tried alternative treatments like homeopathy and acupuncture. Despite all of this, his back hurts so badly that he cannot sit or stand for long periods of time. It doesn't take a rocket scientist to know that the body's natural healing processes are unlikely to improve the situation. His back is probably as good as it is going to get. That being so, it is safe to diagnose this patient as having the medical condition known as chronic pain.

 From the Doctor's Journal:

In my practice, "Millie," a retired nurse, holds the record for duration of chronic pain. She was in her 70's when she came to see me, and told me that she had suffered from pain in her buttocks for

68

more than fifty years. As I write about her case now, I see the temptation people might feel to make a cute joke about the location and duration of her pain. But there was nothing funny about the suffering of the woman who sat before me in my exam room telling me the long, tragic saga of her pain.

My mind reeled when she talked about her medical history. As she told me about the doctors she had seen and the interventions she had had over a half century, I thought about what else had been occurring at that time. When she first saw a doctor for her problem, I was in diapers. As she ticked off the events of her illness, I thought, that was when Eisenhower had his heart attack...that was when Kennedy was shot...that was when the astronauts landed on the moon.

Of all the medicines over all the years, the only one that had done her any good at all was a combination of hydrocodone and acetaminophen. That was somewhat better than no medicine at all, but not much. And I could not simply raise the dose since a significant increase in the dosage of acetaminophen would expose her to the risk of liver damage.

I decided to treat her with a pure opioid, so that I could safely raise the dose. I tried her on sustained-release oxycodone, to no avail. It made her feel nauseated and woozy. Sustained-release morphine did the same. I then tried low dose transcutaneous fentanyl, and was surprised and pleased to learn that she tolerated it, even though it did little for her pain. I gradually increased the dose, escalating from patches of 25 micrograms (mcg.) per hour to 50, and again to 75. Then, the patient and her observant son noticed a strange phenomenon. Millie would wear her patch for three days, as instructed. On the first day, she would be too sleepy to get out of bed. On the second day, she felt good, energetic, and with little pain. On the third day, she was alert, but the buttock pain was bothering her.

I realized that Millie's problem was irregular absorption of the medicine from the patch. For Millie, the amount of drug in the blood stream had to be *just so* or it would either cause side effects or be ineffective.

With the help of her keen observation—there is an advantage to having a nurse as a patient—I was able to devise a plan for her. I asked Millie to wear three patches at a time, each one being 25 mcg. per hour. She would replace one of them daily, so that she had one patch in its first day of being worn, one in its second day, and one in its third day. The excessive absorption of the fresh patch was balanced by the feeble absorption from the oldest patch. This smoothed out the absorption of the drug, and, for the first time since Harry Truman strode through the Rose Garden, Millie was free of her gnawing pain.

When dealing with chronic pain, we can rely on the fact that *without* treatment the pain is simply not going to disappear. That is all the more reason to attack the condition—or dis-ease, if you will—aggressively in order to burst through the barriers to effective chronic pain control and bring desperately needed relief.

The Barriers to Effective Chronic Pain Control

We have good news and bad news, and good news and bad news again. The good news is that chronic pain is substantially controllable. In other words, medical science knows how to bring substantial relief in almost all cases. The bad news is that there are numerous roadblocks between pain and its effective palliation. The good news is that physicians and patients can surmount these obstacles. It just takes grit, determination, and a willingness to keep trying until the job is done. The bad news, alas, is that too many doctors and patients quit trying to access relief before they truly run out of options.

Roadblock # 1: The Use of the Wrong Medicine

Too many doctors prescribe and too many patients receive the wrong therapy to treat chronic pain. For example, many patients take nonsteroidal anti-inflammatory drugs (NSAIDs, see Chapter 3), such as aspirin or ibuprofen, for many years, even if they receive little benefit from the medication. Not only do they continue to have uncontrolled pain, but they face a cumulative risk of serious adverse effects of these drugs. In 1998, Dr. G. Singh published data in the *American Journal of Medicine* showing that over 16,000 NSAID-related deaths occur each year among arthritis patients alone. This is greater than the number of Americans who die of AIDS.

Other chronic pain sufferers receive pathetically inadequate doses of weak opioids in combination with acetaminophen (Tylenol®). While these hybrid drugs might be fine for moderate or for intermittent pain, they are usually just not strong enough for chronic pain that is moderate to severe. Indeed, they may do more harm than good, giving just enough relief to keep the patient taking them (and from seeking more effective relief), but not enough to restore the patient to a truly active life.

Roadblock # 2: "As Needed" Prescriptions

Many physicians instruct their patients to take their pain medication on an "as needed" basis. (Doctors call as-needed prescriptions "prn," which is simply a Latin abbreviation for "as-needed.") In other words, the patient is to take the medicine only when the pain becomes so bad that he or she has no other choice. For most chronic pain patients, that occurs several times per day, every day, week after week, month after month, year after miserable year. And every leap year simply offers an extra day of pain. This is a misguided approach to controlling chronic pain. "As needed" prescriptions may actually *hinder* rather than help effective palliation, because the patient isn't likely to take the medicine until he or she is really hurting. In other words, the pain gets ahead of the medicine, which makes it more difficult for the medicine to do its work effectively.

If we really want to control chronic pain, we must keep the pain-causing network permanently off the air, rather than try to shut it down once it begins broadcasting. Think about this for a moment, and compare the way many doctors prescribe for chronic pain with the way they prescribe for other chronic health conditions. For example, do doctors treat diabetes by prescribing insulin "as needed for diabetic coma"? Of course not. That would be medical malpractice. We know that diabetics must take their insulin before the symptoms of dangerously high blood sugar begin to appear. Similarly, we don't treat high blood pressure by saying, "Take this pill as needed for congestive heart failure or stroke." On the contrary, the drugs are prescribed to prevent the illness from advancing to the point where symptoms or complications occur. There is no reason why chronic pain should be approached any differently.

To treat chronic pain with only "as needed" therapy, guarantees that the therapy will fail. Rather than being treated prn, chronic pain should be treated around-the-clock (ATC) to prevent the pain from taking hold in the first place. That is one meaning of the term "power over pain."

Roadblock # 3: Misunderstanding Morphine

So much pain is caused by the myths about morphine that we devoted much of the last chapter to the subject. But, since this issue is so important, the truths about morphine bear repeating:

72

- Properly prescribed and taken, morphine is safe;

- Morphine used for pain control is not addicting;

- Increasing dosage to match increasing pain is safe;

- Using morphine for today's pain does not mean it will not work on tomorrow's pain;

- Increased dosage requirements do not necessarily mean that one is dying;

- Properly used, morphine does not cause stupor.

The underutilization of opioids is one of this country's great silent tragedies, and we, at least, intend to be silent no longer. As we shall see below, morphine and other opioids are excellent medicines for chronic pain. If you are in chronic pain and require morphine or other such medicines, don't let the myths about morphine fool you or your doctor into underutilizing this marvelous treatment.

Roadblock # 4: Pain is Not Taken Seriously

As mentioned above, in this country pain is treated as if it were somehow different from other "real" diseases. If pain were a person, it would be plain to see that it is treated with nothing short of shocking and shameful bigotry. And since pain is not an abstract concept, but something very real that can diminish or even destroy lives, the ultimate victims of this bigotry are suffering people.

In spite of the fact that one of the most common health problems in America is chronic pain, doctors often claim that they're "not comfortable" treating such pain with the class of drugs most effective in its management. Pharmacies interrogate patients carrying prescriptions for opioids, humiliating them publicly in front of other customers. Mail-order pharmacies routinely diminish the number of tablets sent to a patient despite the written prescription of the doctor because "too many" have been prescribed. They would certainly not limit the number of units of insulin dispensed to a diabetic patient, or the dose of a medicine to treat high blood pressure. But for some reason, pain is different. In most states, Medicaid programs routinely deny access to adequate quantities of opioid medication unless a time-consuming phone call is made to a bureaucratic minion in a far-away city who—without ever having met the patient and without a medical degree—must "approve" the prescription.

Roadblock # 5: Physicians Not Trained to Treat Chronic Pain

The problem is not simply that doctors are not trained to treat chronic pain. It is worse than that. They are often mistrained. The fact that medical school education in pain control is deficient is unarguable. But that, in itself, is not catastrophic. Most real medical education occurs after medical school, but pain-control training during the post-graduate years—the time in a doctor's education when it matters most—is abysmal. It is a case of the blind leading the blind: most of the doctors who teach the residents are themselves ignorant of the advances in pain medicine.

Moreover, young doctors absorb the medical culture where it is often assumed that treatment of pain is a secondary issue. The chief surgeon will see to it that the stitch is tied just so, but then, after the operation, will turn to the chief resident and say, "Write an order for some pain medicine." The chief resident will turn to the junior resident, passing along the same order. The junior resident will give it to the intern, who is less than a year out of school. If he does not turn over the job to a medical student, he'll simply write whatever medication he has learned about from his on-call buddy, or the resident who preceded him.

Adding to the problem, many training hospitals are located in poor urban neighborhoods. Patients who frequent their outpatient clinics, where post-graduate doctors train, are usually poor, powerless, and often don't follow the instructions for taking their medicine. (This is a problem that is certainly not restricted to the poor or less

74

educated.) These patients have no private doctor, despite the fact that many have Medicaid insurance—and there are doctors who accept such patients. But patients who go to training clinics often have not been able to "connect" with a private doctor. Sometimes it is due to transportation problems, but other times it is because of drug abuse, alcoholism, or personal negligence. Consequently, patients who are "teaching cases" for young doctors are a select group, not at all representative of patients in general or of poor patients in particular. Those in charge of training fledgling doctors warn them not to believe the patients, to doubt their complaints of pain, because so many, they say, are drug abusers trying to "hustle" naive young doctors. This lesson is learned all too well, so that the doctors ever after are dubious about complaints of chronic pain, especially if the patient is poor, non-elderly, African-American, or Latino.

 ### *From the Doctor's Journal:*

Of course, drug users and criminals are not immune to chronic pain. In fact, they are more likely than others to develop the condition because their risky life styles expose them to more illness and trauma. But woe to them when they do, for their complaints are seldom believed. A recent patient of mine exemplifies the troubles they may have, and I am sobered to realize how many such people I may have inadequately treated in years past.

When I first met him, I thought that "James" had just about everything going against him. He was poor, black, disabled, and, according to the emergency room doctor, "crazy." The ER doctor sent him to the psychiatric unit for fear that he was suicidal or even homicidal. An even greater impediment to his treatment, however, was the fact that James was—how shall I put this—woefully short on social skills. Whenever he was frustrated by inadequate or dismissive treatment, which was fairly often, he would respond with anger and threats to his doctors.

Yet James' pain was real and severe. He had suffered a spinal cord injury in what newspapers would call "a drug deal gone bad." The bullet had not completely transected his spinal cord, so he was still able to walk. But his gait was severely stooped and spastic, that is, he could not straighten his legs well and, when he tried to walk, they crossed over each other like the blades of a scissors.

His back and leg pain had been present for several years when I met him. A neurosurgeon had implanted a pump and spinal catheter into him. That had helped a little for a while, but the pump was now empty because all the neurosurgeons in town refused to take care of him.

I was not very optimistic when I began to treat him. The key to caring for a patient, it has been remarked, is to *care* for the patient. Try as I did, there was, at first, little in James that I found likable. Still, he was a man suffering from chronic pain, and I could not simply write him off.

I started by treating the spasticity. I felt that some of his pain was consequent to the muscle spasms, and that treating the spasticity could improve both the pain and the gait disturbance. Not a secondary consideration was the fact that treating the spasticity could be accomplished without use of controlled substances, which I feared he was likely to abuse.

When James' gait improved, it was like a fog beginning to lift. I saw the first glimmer of some likeability in his character. For the first time, I sensed that he was speaking to me without deception. He freely mentioned that he was still using heroin on occasion, an admission that no savvy drug hustler would ever make to a doctor.

Still, I was not confident that James could use oral opioids without abusing them, or, which would be as bad, without my suspecting him of abusing them. I felt that fentanyl (Duragesic®) delivered across the skin would be a better medicine for him. It's an easy drug to monitor. You just ask the patient to show you the patch on his skin. I knew that a sophisticated junkie could extract and inject the fentanyl from the patch, but James was not that sophisticated, and I felt that the potential benefit of the medicine exceeded the potential for harm to him.

Because of the long-lasting severity of his pain, and because he was likely to be somewhat tolerant to opioids due to his prior drug abuse, I expected him to need a relatively high dose of fentanyl to achieve adequate pain relief. I was prepared for him to complain that the initial low dose was inadequate, and I consciously planned not to interpret demands for a higher dose as a sign of abuse. But to my surprise, James achieved substantial and satisfactory pain relief from the lowest dose of the patch. There were no telltale signs of drug abuse or diversion. He did not "lose" his prescriptions. The dog did not eat them. In plain language, there was simply no hustle. Instead I now saw a man who could walk with his head held high—both literally and figuratively.

The challenge now is to find a surgeon willing to remove the pump that he no longer needs, and perhaps never did. I'm working on that. James is already participating fully in physical therapy, improving his gait further now that the pain is controlled. The final phase of his therapy will be vocational rehabilitation. Time will tell, but perhaps now that his pain is under control, James will be able to address his dysfunctional life.

Roadblock #6: Pain Is Not Recognized As a Distinct Disease

Regrettably, doctors are trained to see pain as a symptom requiring explanation, that is, as a valuable clue leading to a diagnosis, rather than as a disease in its own right. It is still standard teaching in surgery training programs to avoid treating a patient's acute abdominal pain lest the treatment mask the cause of the illness producing the pain. While that may or may not be an appropriate approach for acute abdominal pain (there is some evidence that the classical teaching is wrong), it is certainly completely wrong-headed in the case of chronic pain. For many chronic pain patients, we cannot figure out exactly why they have pain. The "failed back patient" (notice that the doctors do not refer to them as "failed surgery patients") often has X-rays and physical findings indistinguishable from patients who benefited from the surgery. Almost all chronic headache patients have normal brain scans. So the doctor says, "I can't find out what's the problem"—and then does nothing!

It does not have to be this way. Doctors treat many diseases whose cause is unknown, often using therapies whose mechanisms of action are similarly mysterious. For example, doctors usually cannot explain the cause of high blood pressure. The cause of obesity, similarly, remains a mystery and is the subject of ongoing research. Yet both of these diseases are recognized and treated, with varying success, every day. Why should pain be any different? Just as high blood pressure *may* be a symptom of an underlying disease (such as narrowing of the artery leading to the kidney), so pain *may* be a symptom of a definable and treatable condition. But when it is not, pain should be treated as vigorously as any other medical condition with an unknown origin.

Similarly, when a medication is useful to relieve a symptom, it should be used even if the way it works is unclear. It was hundreds of years before medical scientists understood how morphine worked. At the time of this writing, the precise mechanism that enables many drugs to successfully treat nerve pain remains undefined. Still, there is no reason to wait for every question to be answered before proceeding to enjoy the benefits that effective therapies offer.

Getting the Job Done

The best medicine for moderate to severe chronic pain is usually morphine, oxycodone, or some other opioid. At one time it was believed that these medicines work only in the treatment of nociceptive (tissue damage) pain, such as that caused by cancer, but that they are not useful in the management of neuropathic (nerve damage) pain, a frequent cause of chronic pain. In fact, opioids are of potential benefit in both types of pain. However, neuropathic pain often requires doses of opioids higher than those needed for tissue damage pain. This can cause a real problem for patients with nerve pain, since the myths about morphine may inhibit the physician from prescribing and the patient from taking the necessary dose.

This is not to say that taking morphine or other opioids is as simple as the doctor saying, "Take two aspirin and call me in the morning." These are drugs that require knowledgeable prescribing and careful management. Fortunately, there are a number of imaginative ways to deliver opioids that permit effective relief in most cases.

The Importance of Time

At this point in our discussion, we need to describe a characteristic of morphine and other opioids that is important to understanding the proper use of these medicines: the length of time they are effective in the body. Most readers will have heard of the term "half-life" as a way of describing the length of time a radioactive material will continue to emit radiation. Thus, a radioactive material with a half-life of five years will have given off half of its radioactivity in that time. In the next five years, it will again yield half of its remaining radioactivity. Put differently, if you start with a pound of radioactive material with a half-life of five years, then you will have half a pound of radioactive material at the end of five years, and a quarter pound of it at the end of ten years, and an eighth of a pound of it at the end of fifteen years, etc.

Half-life is a term that is also applied to medicine. A half-life of a drug refers to how long it takes the body to remove half of the drug from the blood stream. It is one measure of how long the beneficial effect of the drug will persist. There are rare exceptions, but, in general, a drug with a long half-life has a longer duration of action, and, therefore, will require less frequent dosing. It is important to know how long your pain control medicine is expected to exert its pain-relieving effect. That will help you understand how often to take it.

Not all opioids have the same half-life, and, consequently, they have widely varying durations of action. Plain old morphine taken by mouth usually yields pain relief lasting about four hours. So one way that morphine can be given is every four hours, *by the clock*, to prevent pain. Although this works, it is inconvenient. If the patient fails to set the alarm clock to get up in the middle of the night to take the scheduled dose, he or she will likely awaken in severe pain. The result is not simply agony, but also greater difficulty in getting the pain back under control.

Fortunately, we now have available several different opioids that have been formulated to yield long-acting pain relief. Most of these achieve the effect by being absorbed slowly from the medicine vehicle. "Pain control vehicle" means the kind of delivery system by which the medicine gets into the body. Usually, this will be a pill. But the vehicle can be a patch that delivers medicine across the skin continuously, or a pump that is implanted into the body allowing the patient to receive a continuous flow of the medicine.

Morphine, as just one example, is available in sustained-release tablets that yield up their contents over twelve or twenty-four hours. Trade names of these morphine products include MS-Contin®, Oramorph-SR®, and Kadian®. Other brands will doubtless become available in the future.

An example of a non-morphine opioid that lasts over time is OxyContin®, the trade name of a long-acting tablet that contains the opioid oxycodone. It lasts twelve hours for most patients. Recently, this drug has received a fair bit of notoriety because of some well-publicized cases of its purposeful misuse by drug addicts. The addicts grind up the drug and snort it or inject it, often with a variety of other drugs, in an effort to overcome the slow-release mechanism that the pharmaceutical scientists had worked so hard to create. Some of these cases resulted in the deaths of those who intentionally abused the drug. Of course, this rare misuse of the drug should not deter its proper use, as directed by a knowledgeable physician, in appropriate patients. In the near future, a 24-hour formulation of the opioid hydromorphone may join the list of available long-acting opioids.

Yet another opioid, fentanyl, would be a particularly short-acting drug if it were just taken by mouth. But when it is formulated as Duragesic®, a patch whose contents are absorbed over 48-72 hours, it can provide long-lasting pain relief. (This list is not exclusive, nor are we endorsing any single brand.) You may wish to ask your doctor about these and other long-term opioid medicines.

The benefits of time-release pain medicine are obvious. Pain can be kept under continuous control. Patients don't have to interrupt their sleep to ensure that they awaken pain free and ready to tackle the day. Life can be lived with the minimal amount of disruption caused by chronic pain.

Finally, there are some opioids whose intrinsic half-life is long enough to preclude the need for slow-release formulation. Methadone belongs to this category. Methadone, of course, has achieved recognition because it is also used to treat some kinds of drug addiction. Unfortunately, this has led some patients to identify methadone as "a drug for junkies." This is a shame, because it is a perfectly useful opioid, and a relatively inexpensive one. Here's an analogy: penicillin may be used to treat syphilis, and it may also be used to treat pneumonia. That does not make penicillin a "drug for syphilitics" any more than its use to treat drug addiction makes methadone a "drug for junkies."

From the Doctor's Journal:

Sometimes, the stigma of methadone affects the thinking even of savvy doctors. A psychiatrist colleague of mine asked me to see a patient of his who was having trouble withdrawing from methadone. The patient, I was told, was a man in his 60s who had developed a "drug problem" while being treated for chronic pain from multiple injuries. He had gone through an expensive and, from my viewpoint, horrific "rapid detoxification program" at a nearby referral center, but he had done poorly afterward. The psychiatrist had then put him on methadone to treat what appeared to be ongoing withdrawal symptoms, but the doctor was stymied in his attempts to taper the drug. Whenever he lowered the dose below a certain threshold, the patient would deteriorate physically, and become depressed, even suicidal.

I evaluated the patient in my office. He was a somber, somewhat irritable man, who said that he sincerely wanted to stop taking drugs, but he felt miserable whenever he tried to reduce the dose. As I probed his story in more detail, I learned that the misery he experienced was *not* that of withdrawal symptoms, but rather, the recurrence of his pain.

My advice came as a surprise to the patient. I didn't want him to take less methadone, but more. He was having no side effects from the drug, nor was he addicted. (Remember the quick definition of addiction: use despite harm. His harm was not coming from using the drug; it was coming from stopping it.) He had achieved partial remission of his pain on methadone, but he had never really taken enough to get truly satisfactory pain relief.

At my instruction, he raised his methadone dose—and became a new man. No longer somber or irritable, certainly no longer suicidal, he came to the office smiling and joyously relating the activities he could now do that had once seemed to be foreclosed to him forever. Before proper treatment, he had barely been able to get out of the house. Now he had returned to his hobby of "working horses." True, he could not ride horses as he had before his injuries, but he could lead them through the corral by their reins and do some simple chores around the barn.

The patient had felt that, because he was taking methadone, he was a drug addict, and, for that reason, he had been eager to stop taking the medicine. The psychiatrist had been misled by the fact that the patient had come to see him after failed therapy for drug addiction. No wonder the drug addiction therapy had failed. The wrong disease was being treated. This patient wasn't a drug addict.

Some peculiarities of methadone preclude it from being the drug of choice for most doctors to prescribe, but when prescribed by knowledgeable physicians who understand these intricacies, it can yield remarkably good pain relief. The doctor prescribing methadone must understand that a long half-life also means that the drug can accumulate in the blood stream over the first few days of the patient's taking it. Therefore, doses cannot be changed as rapidly with methadone as with other opioids. Other technical features of dose calculation, when converting a patient from morphine or oxycodone to methadone, make it a drug for only experienced clinicians to prescribe. But, despite these challenges, it is still an underused drug.

The Rhythms of Chronic Pain

If pain intensity were unchanging during the day, then uniform, around the clock dosing would be sufficient for its control. However, pain, like the tide, ebbs and flows in intensity. Some of this phenomenon is due to the natural rhythm of the bodily functions, and some due to the variations of pain-inducing activity in which patients engage during the day. Many patients experience variation in pain intensity depending on the weather. And sometimes chronic pain flares for no apparent reason.

When pain "breaks through" the control achieved through the proper use of ATC (around-the-clock) medication, it should not be ignored or worked around, but treated, as instructed by your doctor, on an "as needed" basis. Of course, if too many breakthroughs occur during the day, that is a signal to the patient and the doctor that the current dose of the ATC opioid may need to be increased. How many pain breakthroughs are too many? Most doctors say more than three or four such episodes warrant an increase in the around-the-clock dose. But keep in mind that the goal of therapy is patient satisfaction with pain control. Most people prefer to have as few as possible episodes of breakthrough pain. But others feel more "in control" if they experience a breakthrough episode and can then repeatedly demonstrate that they can control it. If the patient is content with the number of breakthrough episodes and their control, well, mission accomplished.

When All Else Fails, Be Creative

So far, we have seen that chronic pain is a medical condition that usually can be treated successfully with standard forms of pain therapy.

84

But that is not true in every case. There are some forms of chronic pain that are so intractable that they require reinforcements equivalent to the cavalry riding to the rescue. These kinds of treatments are known as "advanced therapy systems" (ATS).

In general, ATS interventions are reserved for cases of chronic pain for which the usual treatments are ineffective and/or in which the intensity of side effects make them unusable. It is theoretically possible that these ATS interventions are really preferable, that they actually should be resorted to first rather than last. But that is a matter for ongoing research. For now, since there is no real evidence supporting that theory and since these interventions carry greater cost and health risk because they require surgery, ATS treatments are reserved for those cases requiring creative measures.

Spinal Pumps

You will recall from Chapter 4 that opioids exert a good deal of their pain-controlling effect in the spinal cord, where the drug blocks the pain signal. But when the drug is taken orally, via patch, or even intravenously, the effects will also be felt elsewhere in the body, such as by causing a slowing of the workings of the intestines, leading to constipation.

Fortunately, most people can adjust to these side effects, either with the passage of time, or by the use of medication to reduce their intensity. But what happens if a patient gets good pain relief from the medicine, but only at the price of intractable and intolerable side effects, such as severe sedation? Then we would want to deliver morphine to the spinal cord and not to the brain. In that way, the benefit would be achieved with fewer of the burdens

In practice, we cannot deliver the opioid *only* to the spinal cord, but we can deliver it *primarily* to that site. A slender tube (catheter) can be inserted into the fluid that bathes the spinal cord, or just outside the membrane that surrounds the spinal cord. In this way, the medicine can be delivered through the catheter on a continuous basis. The opioid is now in high concentration where it is needed most—in the region of the spinal cord—but in much lower levels elsewhere, leading to good pain control and substantially reduced side effects. Another reason for the diminished side effects is that the amount of medicine needed to control pain is much lower. One beauty of the spinal catheter is that pain-controlling drugs other than opioids can also be delivered via this route. The local anesthetic lidocaine, and its longer-acting near relative bupivicaine, may be infused through the spinal pump as well.

Most of us think of lidocaine as the drug the dentist uses to make our gums numb during dental procedures. Lidocaine, used this way by a dentist, is not technically a pain-controlling drug. Rather, it is an anesthetic because it does not simply prevent pain; it blocks *all* sensation. That may be useful when a small area of the body, say, the gums or a patch of skin, is to be treated. Even then, it is really only useful on a temporary basis. Thus, lidocaine would seem to be an unlikely candidate for spinal therapy, since we certainly don't want anesthesia! After all, we want to be able to feel our legs.

Fortunately, lidocaine and bupivicaine in low concentration interfere mainly with pain sensation, while allowing other sensations to travel the nerves to the spinal cord. By themselves, these local anesthetics are only modestly useful agents in spinal therapy. *But when administered along with an opioid*, they can significantly enhance the analgesic effect. Their side effects are predictable. If too high a concentration is used, or if the patient is extraordinarily sensitive to the usual concentration of the drug, the result may be numbness or weakness in the legs and pelvis, and possibly temporary loss of control of bladder and bowel function.

Another drug that should soon become available for intraspinal use is ziconitide. (At the time of this writing, the drug has achieved FDA approval for marketing, but is not yet available.) This unusual drug is derived from the venom of a Pacific sea snail. Its mechanism of action is completely different from that of other agents used spinally, and has been shown to be useful in even some of the most treatment-resistant cases of chronic pain. Since it is not effective when taken orally or intravenously, it must be used via the spinal catheter.

Finally, we should not ignore clonidine. This drug has been used for many years to treat high blood pressure. Its pain-relieving action at doses tolerable by mouth is negligible. The oral dose needed for significant pain relief would be intolerable because it would make the blood pressure drop to hazardous levels. But when used by injection directly into the spinal fluid, it can reverse pain with significantly less impact on the blood pressure. Some clinicians feel that clonidine is even a better agent than morphine for intraspinal use. Expect to hear more about this old drug via this new route in the future.

Ideally, a spinal catheter should first be implanted on a temporary basis, to prove that the patient can benefit from the drug administered through it. After that is proven, the system can be made permanent. To make the system permanent requires minor surgery. Under anesthesia, the catheter is tunneled under the skin from where it leaves the spine to the front flank of the abdomen. The surgeon then creates a pocket under the skin for the implantation of a small battery operated pump to attach to the catheter. The pump is filled with medicine when it is implanted, and later it may be refilled via a hypodermic needle across the skin. In the small group of patients for whom non-surgical therapies have failed, this can give very satisfactory pain relief on a long-term basis.

Clearly, this procedure is not for everyone. It makes no sense to use a spinal catheter if the drug can be taken safely with less invasive methods, since there are some downsides to this procedure. But people who need this level of medical treatment are generally so desperate that the minor risks are clearly worth the hoped-for benefit.

The most important surgical risks are complications of anesthesia (these are thankfully rare), infection, and bleeding. These risks with this procedure are not prohibitive, and are probably lower than similar risks with an appendectomy or tonsillectomy. Even after the pump has been in place for a long period of time, there is an ongoing, albeit tiny, risk of infection, in much the same way as people who have had a hip replacement or other prosthesis implanted in the body remain at some risk of infection. In such cases, common sense and ordinary precautions should prevent most trouble. For example, just as patients who have had a hip replacement are well advised to take antibiotics before dental procedures to avoid possible infection, patients who have a pump in place should inform their dentists about it, since most dentists will want to prescribe an antibiotic prior to any dental work.

A more irritating downside to the procedure is that the pump needs ongoing attention. We don't simply put it in and forget about it. The pump will need to be refilled from time to time. The frequency of that need depends, of course, on the dose the patient is receiving. The dose or even choice of the analgesic medication may change over time. Every few years the batteries wear out, and then the pump must be replaced. This requires minor surgery.

Some readers, at this point, will begin to worry about the cost of implanted pumps. In general, external pumps are cheaper than implanted ones for short-term use, but more expensive when used for more than a few months. So, an implanted pump system, while it costs more than oral opioids, can actually be cost effective long term, at least when compared to the use of a spinal catheter connected to an external pump. For patients who will have the pump in place for more than a few months, the permanent (implanted) pump system represents a cost savings when compared with inserting a spinal catheter but leaving the pump external to the body.

However, terminally ill patients who need spinal therapy are more likely to benefit from it when it is delivered via an external pump. These patients are usually in a poor position to tolerate the insertion of a permanent pump, which requires surgery, as opposed to a catheter insertion, which can be done via a mere needle stick. Here the cost saving is a side benefit, but does not drive the decision-making.

Ironically, many insurance policies, as well as Medicare, will pay for the implantation and servicing of a spinal therapy pump, but will not pay for oral pain medications taken by patients outside of a hospital or hospice setting. This is truly an example of "penny wise and pound foolish." In some cases, the spinal therapy actually provides considerable financial relief (for the patient, not the insurance company or government) as well as pain relief.

Spinal Cord Stimulators

The second kind of advanced therapy system also involves a spinal device, but is really quite different from spinal drug delivery pumps. It is called a spinal cord stimulator (SCS). It is also occasionally referred to as a dorsal column stimulator. An SCS is an electrode that is placed under the skin and directly over the part of the spinal cord that is communicating the chronic pain information to the brain. For patients with low back and leg pain, this is usually the lumbar spinal cord, the lowest part of the cord.

Electricity from the stimulator directly affects the cells in the spinal cord, causing them to send a message to the brain. The patient feels a tingling or buzzing sensation, but that sure beats pain! While the spinal cord is busy sending this tingling or buzzing information to the brain, its capacity to send pain information is reduced. The stimulator works by exchanging the pain message with a far less onerous one. The patient may be in "tingle" but will be substantially out of pain.

It is important to distinguish this technology from TENS (transdermal electrical nerve stimulation). In TENS therapy, an electrode is applied to the skin to stimulate a nerve far from the spinal cord. The cord itself is never directly stimulated with TENS. In SCS, by contrast, only the cord is stimulated. TENS has some usefulness in mild to moderate pain, but is seldom beneficial when pain is moderate to severe in intensity. SCS may be useful even in these most difficult cases, but is too invasive to be warranted in treatment of pain of only mild to moderate intensity.

The implantation of a permanent spinal cord stimulator is usually preceded by the insertion of a temporary electrical lead to accomplish the same purpose. It is important to be sure that the catheter can be placed over the appropriate level of the spinal cord, and that the location of buzzing can "cover" the area of pain. Most importantly, the patient must decide if the buzzing feeling (which most describe as mildly annoying at worst) is tolerable and preferable to the prior pain.

The implanted spinal cord stimulator electrode must be connected to a power source; otherwise it is a dead wire. Compact batteries, similar to cardiac pacemakers, are available for this purpose. They are implanted under the skin on the side of the abdomen or high in the buttocks, in a manner similar to that of spinal cord pumps. Like pumps, they have a limited life span, and must be replaced every few years when the battery wears out.

This chapter has informed you of the various types of treatments available for severe chronic pain. It is not intended to take the place of your physician, but can be of tremendous use to you in discussing with your doctor the approaches to try if simpler approaches to pain control prove ineffective. Additionally, if your doctor is unfamiliar with these treatment therapies, the time has probably come to ask for a referral to a pain control specialist.

Maybe your doctor would appreciate a copy of this book, too!

CHAPTER 6

■

Treating Acute Pain

Most people believe that the word "acute" means severe. It does not. "Acute" pain can be severe or minor. When describing pain, the word acute, like the word chronic, actually refers to the pain's expected duration. Acute pain, generally stated, is pain of short duration—be it the minor ouch of a paper cut or the agony of being stabbed in the abdomen.

How briefly must pain persist to qualify as acute pain? Here we go again with the definitions. In pain medicine, acute pain is sometimes defined as pain lasting for less than six months. Other researchers define it as pain due to a surgical procedure or bodily injury. One textbook simply defines it as the mirror opposite of our definition of chronic pain, that is, as pain that is likely to get better by itself without treatment.

All of this reminds us of the old story of the blind men and the elephant. When asked to describe the beast, the first man grabs its tail and says it is like a snake. The next one touches its leg and says it is akin to a tree, and so on. All may be true and yet incomplete. However, since this is not a medical textbook or a research paper written for publication in a medical journal, we'll leave the explicit definitions behind, confident that you understand the type of pain we are dealing with in this chapter.

Acute pain has a different meaning, both to doctor and to the patient, than does chronic pain. A comparison will explain why. As we write this chapter, we are both in our early fifties. Over the last five years, one of us has grown fairly bald, the other fairly gray. The little bit of thinning or dusting of gray that once was barely noticeable is now quite pronounced on our respective heads. This "hair evolution" proceeded gradually and expectedly as a natural part of aging. Thus, while the reminders in our mirrors that life is a one-way street may not have especially pleased us, at least we were not alarmed when our hair ceased to appear youthful. Sure, we grumbled to our barbers, but neither of us went to the doctor to find out if anything was wrong.

But what if our hair had grown bald or silver overnight? Rather than merely being a matter of vanity, such a sudden and unexpected change in our bodies would indicate a potentially serious health problem. In such a case, calling our doctors for an immediate appointment would be the first order of business for the day.

Sudden pain where none existed before is—and should be—extremely alarming. The person with new pain recognizes that there must be a reason why a part of his or her body hurts. Very often, worried patients will explain to the doctor that the pain itself is not so severe as to require treatment, but its *presence* is the problem, because it implies undiagnosed disease. A good doctor recognizes that the patient's acute pain is often a clue to the presence and identity of an illness, and the doctor will use the details of the pain to guide the diagnostic workup.

Acute pain also causes anxiety for another reason. Our brains are actually programmed to experience acute pain as an anxiety-provoking experience. Although we like to think of ourselves as rational creatures, a large part of our brain is dedicated to the perception and regulation of emotions. As touched upon earlier in this book, part of the information concerning pain is sent from the spinal cord to the part of the brain that mediates the experience of emotion. It is only a slight exaggeration to say that the essence of acute pain is as much the anxiety provoked by the painful stimulus, as it is the physical discomfort of the pain. It is a foolish doctor, indeed, who attributes the acute pain of an anxious patient to the anxiety itself.

As we have seen, acute pain can cause a patient to seek medical help in the hope of finding the pain's cause and a remedy for it. Occasionally, however, the opposite may occur. Patients with cancer, especially those whose disease has been in remission, fear that every new ache or pain is a sure sign that the cancer has come back. Not wanting to face that possibility, they will downplay the intensity of the pain, claiming it's really "no big deal," even if the pain is fairly disabling. While some of these patients do indeed have a relapse of the cancer, many do not. One of the first lessons that oncologists learn is that pain experienced by cancer patients is not necessarily cancer pain. After all, having cancer is no immunization against shingles, arthritis, tennis elbow, appendicitis, or any other painful condition.

Controlling Acute Pain

The first task in managing acute pain, logically, is to find out why it hurts. This is not as easy as it sounds. Similar pain can be caused by a wide variety of ailments. Thus, the doctor will first determine, with as much precision as possible, the location and extent of the pain. Then, if the cause is not readily apparent, diagnostic tests will be conducted. These tests serve two purposes: first, since the art of diagnosis is often a "ruling out" enterprise, an important part of medical testing is finding out what is *not* causing the pain. Then, the scope of the search is narrowed to determine the pain's cause so it can be treated. After that, the acute pain itself will be treated, either in connection with treating the cause or, if necessary, before the diagnosis is complete.

Most acute conditions that cause pain are treatable. Cuts may be stitched, broken bones set, infections treated with antibiotics, and inflamed appendices cut out. Then, both doctor and patient wait while nature gets about the work of healing the injury, which eventually ends the acute pain.

Acute pain is almost always associated with what doctors call inflammation and most people call swelling. Inflammation is characterized by the presence of *rubor, dolor, calor*, and *lassio functionis*. For those of you who did not brush up on your Latin this morning, that is redness, pain, heat, and loss of function. Whenever the body experiences some injury or other sudden physical disorder, the immune system gets busy secreting a veritable stew of chemicals at that site. These chemicals are called the mediators of inflammation. As discussed in Chapter 3, they cause blood vessels to dilate to allow the immune system to do its work efficiently. First, the increased flow of blood caused by the blood vessel expansion allows better access to the site for more white blood cells and other components of the immune system. The increased blood flow raises the temperature of the injury site, and changes its color to red. It also allows some swelling to occur at that area, diminishing flexibility. This is nature's way of constructing a local brace to prevent undue motion that could worsen the injury. The pain itself serves as a powerful reminder and inducement to treat the injured site with care. Thus, when you sprain your ankle, you no longer walk normally, which would increase your injury.

The chemicals are also one of the reasons for pain at the site of acute injury or disease. They rapidly sensitize the pain fibers in the region of the injury, which, as you will recall from Chapter 2, begins the process of transmitting pain information to the brain. These chemicals reduce the level of stimulus necessary to begin the process of feeling pain, as we saw in our earlier example of the sunburned boy playing tag. When the pain nerve fibers are exposed to the chemicals, it takes less of a painful stimulus—less of a squeeze, pinch, or pressure—to trigger the nerves into sending pain signals to the spinal cord and brain. As noted previously, this process is called hyperalgesia.

So, now we know why it hurts and understand that pain is actually part of the healing process. The inflammation associated with pain partially immobilizes the site of injury, and induces the injured

94

person to treat the injury with great care and gentleness. That is fine for times immediately following the injury, or when you cannot get to prompt medical treatment. But with today's medical advances, we no longer need to feel this pain, or at least not so much of it, on an ongoing basis. Indeed, continued severe pain in the face of care, such as surgery, may actually delay healing. Thus, despite the positive aspect of acute pain, there is no reason not to keep its intensity firmly under control.

The first step to treating acute pain is usually treating the injury. This will often include the use of powerful pain control in the form of either local or general anesthesia given during the treatment itself. Unlike opioids and other analgesics, anesthetics cause the loss of all sensation in the parts of the body that are affected. Local anesthesia makes just one part of the body numb. General anesthesia makes the whole body numb by inducing unconsciousness. As an example, if you break your leg, you will receive anesthesia when the doctor sets the bone. Otherwise, you would be in agonizing pain from the act of adjusting the broken bone so it can heal properly. (What an improvement from the days when people undergoing such medical procedures were given a shot of whisky and told to bite down on a rag.)

Because anesthesia stops all sensation in the affected area, it is of limited use as a vehicle for ongoing pain control. That is why, after treating the injury or illness itself, the first step in managing acute pain is to significantly reduce the chemical stew that causes inflammation and its associated pain. Currently there is no drug that eliminates *all* mediators of inflammation, but we do have a large collection of drugs to reduce some of the most important culprits, namely, prostaglandins.

Originally thought to be a single chemical, prostaglandins are, in fact, a family of related chemicals first identified in the male prostate gland. However, despite the name and site of their original discovery, prostaglandins are also found in women.

Prostaglandins are manufactured at sites of inflammation. You might even say that inflammation is manufactured at sites of prostaglandins, since their presence is a cause of the changes we call in-flammation. Drugs that reduce the manufacture of prostaglandins control pain by reducing the sensitization of the pain nerve fibers. That is, they reduce hyperalgesia, and this reduces pain. Fortunately, the drugs do not interfere with the healing purposes of inflammation.

The most commonly used drugs to reduce the manufacture of prostaglandins are the non-steroidal anti-inflammatory drugs (NSAIDs), discussed in Chapter 3. The NSAID with the longest his-tory of clinical use is good old aspirin. Other examples of NSAIDs include ibuprofen (Motrin®), naproxen (Aleve®), and a host of others. These drugs are often adequate to reduce the pain of acute inflamma-tion from a roar to a meow.

When acute pain is moderate to severe in intensity it is usually beyond the ability of NSAIDs to control it. That is the time to call in our old friends the opioids. *It is important to note that the use of morphine or other opioids for treating acute pain should be ap-proached differently than their use in treating chronic pain.* As you will recall, taking morphine or other such medicine on an as needed basis is often inadequate in the treatment of chronic pain. This is because, in the case of chronic pain, we *know* the pain is going to be there unabated, hours, days, and sometimes months from now. In such a case it is important to remain ahead of the pain.

On the other hand, with acute pain we have a different set of circumstances. In acute pain, there are often *rapid changes in the intensity of pain coming from the injured or diseased site.* In such a case, it is reasonable to use opioids as needed for the pain, since there may be significant variation from hour to hour in the pain's intensity. As the injury heals, the pain will likely diminish. Of course, one should not try to "gut it out," enduring pain as long as possible before taking the analgesic. There is no advantage to that at all. To willingly endure pain in the service of a greater cause may be heroic, but to endure pain for no real purpose is no virtue at all.

Surgery is one of the common causes of acute pain that is all too often undertreated. Surgeons are not trained as pain control experts; they are trained as surgeons. Consequently, many do not fully appreciate the value of pain control in postsurgical recovery, and may significantly underestimate how long patients experience pain after going under the knife.

While pain intensity usually subsides within days after surgery, it is far from gone. Often some pain persists for weeks, depending on the extent and the nature of the surgery. This may require a powerful form of pain medicine in the first days after surgery, with a gradual decrease in the strength and type of medicine as time passes, until it is eventually phased out altogether.

Sadly, surgeons often are reluctant to grant patients' requests for ongoing pain control. *"My* operation could not cause so much pain!" the surgeon seems to be saying. A few "negotiating tips" may be in order. *First, be sure to discuss pain control before the surgery.* (Feel free to mention this book. In fact, give the surgeon a copy!) Respectfully tell the surgeon that you expect your pain to be controlled. The doctor will say "of course, of course." *Do not leave it at that.* Ask if you will need morphine after the surgery, or a morphine pump. Inquire whether the surgeon will be willing to continue to control your pain even if it takes longer for you to recover than it does for most patients. If the surgeon hesitates or seems reluctant to meet these basic needs, perhaps you should consider a different surgeon, or receive assurances that a pain control specialist will be consulted if that becomes necessary. More likely, however, your surgeon will promise to do a proper job. Reminding the surgeon of that promise is one way of getting adequate pain relief when the time comes. (It may be advisable to have a spouse, adult child, or other friend or relative come with you to these important discussions to help you communicate effectively about these and other issues of concern. After all, if you are preparing for surgery, you already have plenty on your mind.)

In some cases, however, the patient's request for adequate pain control may take place after the surgery. If your doctor tells you that he or she is "not comfortable prescribing pain pills so long after a surgery" you might respond as follows: "Doctor, I'm sorry that I'm not improving as fast as you had expected, but I'm doing the best I can. What can I do? It still hurts." If the doctor says that it should not be hurting still, you might say, "Yes, it shouldn't be hurting still. But it does. I don't blame you for that, doctor. I hope you won't blame me."

When all else fails, if the surgeon is simply unwilling or unable to control the postoperative pain, simply say, "I appreciate all you've done for me, doctor. I know you've done all you know how to make me feel better. But I'm still in pain. Could you please refer me to a pain control specialist?" This sort of dialogue will either goad the doctor to work harder on pain control out of pride or to happily refer you to someone else just to be rid of you.

Controlling pain after surgery is not only important for your sense of well-being and comfort. It may actually help you heal faster. Studies have shown that surgery patients who receive good pain control often recover more quickly than their counterparts who spend their recuperation period in pain. Thus, pain control is good post-surgical care. The less you are in pain, the sooner you are likely to get on your feet.

 From the Desk of WJS:

A few years ago, when my mother had a hip replacement, I personally witnessed the power of proper pain control to aid the healing process. A hip replacement is potentially a very painful procedure, involving breaking and removing the hipbone and replacing it with a prosthesis. Prior to the surgery, my mother and I spoke at length with her orthopedic surgeon about pain control. "I don't want my mother to have any

98

pain at all," I told him, "or at least any avoidable pain." He said he would do his best to meet this important goal of my mother's treatment.

After the surgery, I visited my mother in her room. She was definitely in no pain, still feeling the effects of the surgical drugs. But she was also attached to an external morphine pump that allowed her to push a button whenever she felt a twinge of pain. The pump is engineered to prevent accidental overdose; it won't inject any morphine if the button is pushed too frequently.

Because my mother was assured by the nurse that she would not receive too much pain control due to the design of the pump, and was assured by me that the use of morphine for this purpose would not cause addiction, she willingly gave herself as much pain control as she needed. As a result, she was able to get on her feet to go to the bathroom sooner than most hip patients, and begin the important process of post-surgical rehabilitation.

When I brought her home, mom was off the pump but on morphine pills for a short time. These were soon replaced by Tylenol® Number Three, a combination drug of Tylenol® and codeine. Soon she was on Tylenol® alone, and then she was off all medicine and pain free.

She had stayed at my place during her convalescence. As she was packing to go back to her own home, mom marveled that she never felt *any* pain during the entire process—from surgery, to hospitalization, to rehabilitation, to recovery. She also appears to have benefited from this important part of her post-surgical care. Her doctor told her that her full recovery came three weeks ahead of schedule.

Most acute pain is caused by injury to the body, like a cut, a broken bone, or other blow to the body. Occasionally, however, neuropathic (nerve) pain may be acute. A good example of this is shingles (also called herpes zoster). Pain may persist for a long time after an attack of shingles, and that is indeed chronic pain. But the skin eruption can also hurt during its first few days. Pain control then is important for two reasons. First, pain control is *always* important. Second, good pain control during the first few days of shingles may reduce the likelihood of the pain becoming chronic.

In 1999 a new formulation of an old drug, the topical anesthetic lidocaine, became available under the trade name Lidoderm® to treat this type of pain. Lidoderm® is a lidocaine-impregnated bandage with an adhesive backing. When put over a site of acute shingles, the patch puts out a steady flow of anesthetic. The dosage is not enough to appear in significant quantity in the blood stream. Therefore, the drug causes no systemic side effects such as general numbness or dizziness. But the lidocaine at the site of the shingles makes that area somewhat sensation free. Within an hour, the patient might notice that there is less pain.

 From the Doctor's Journal:

The importance of controlling the pain of shingles was brought home to me in a personal way. I had just completed treating my father-in-law for a type of lymphoma, a cancer of the lymph nodes, when he developed an outbreak of shingles on the back of his neck. (He has given me permission to discuss his case publicly). Now, my father-in-law is a stoic man, and, at first, said that the blisters on his neck were only annoying, nothing more, really not worth treating. I prescribed an anti-viral medicine for him. Shingles is caused by the same virus that causes chicken pox, and the anti-viral treatment di-

100

minishes the duration of the outbreak. In other words, I treated the cause of the pain but not the pain itself. By the next day, however, he let me know that the pain had worsened significantly, that he had barely slept the night before because of it.

I was eager to avoid using a drug that would cause significant side effects. My father-in-law is over 80 years-old, and even spry alert men such as he are particularly sensitive to the sedating side effects of many analgesics. So, I prescribed Lidoderm® for him, and called him a few hours later to see how he was doing.

It was like talking to a new man. His voice, which had been subdued during the painful episode, sounded energetic. He told me that his pain had completely disappeared within a half hour after applying the Lidoderm®. This was far better than I had expected. Not every patient will get such good results, of course, but this drug, still not known by many doctors, is worth remembering for the treatment of this all too-common condition.

Just as control of side effects is essential for success in the management of chronic pain, it is also essential in the management of acute pain. The challenge is different, however. Over time, the body can adapt to many of the side effects of opioids. On the other hand, the risk of adverse effects of NSAIDs increases with time. Also, the side-effects of treating acute pain are the reverse of those found in management of chronic pain. In acute pain, we do not have time to wait for the body to adjust to opioid side effects. They must be managed aggressively from the very beginning. But, as if to offset this problem, the use of NSAIDs to treat acute pain is seldom complicated by adverse effects.

Sometimes I am asked what the best over-the-counter NSAID is. In truth, there is no best one. For unknown reasons, different people respond better to different agents. Aspirin, ibuprofen, naproxen, ketoprofen are all relatively cheap, safe, and widely available. However, people taking warfarin (Coumadin®) and those with bleeding disorders should not take them without consulting with their doctor. Acetaminophen (Tylenol®), while not an NSAID, is also useful for many cases of mild to moderate pain.

Finally, any chapter on acute pain must ask the question, "When does acute pain become chronic pain?" In some ways, that's like asking when it is that a child becomes an adult. It's easy to recognize when it has happened, but sometimes unclear as to the exact moment when it is happening. If acute pain is not improving after a few weeks or months of its onset, it's likely that it has become chronic. The patient whose pain has evolved from acute to chronic should seek professional advice. Chronic pain need not be intractable pain.

 From the Doctor's Journal:

On rare occasions, a patient may actually need treatment for both acute pain and several types of chronic pain. Such cases present a challenge to the pain physician.

I remember that I was once treating a middle-aged man for two types of chronic pain. He was a diabetic, and, like many diabetics, he had nerve damage in his feet. To make matters worse, he had been born with multiple cysts in his kidneys. Over time, these swelled, causing failure of kidney function. The kidney failure worsened the nerve damage in his feet, and the cysts in the kidney caused pain in the kidneys themselves. Thus, this unfortunate fellow had two types of chronic pain. In his feet, he had neuropathic (nerve damage) pain, while in his flanks he had tissue damage pain. To control these two differ-

102

ent kinds of pain he needed to take a combination of anti-epileptic drugs and the opioid methadone. But with proper dose adjustment, he was able to lead a life limited by his kidney failure, to be sure, but not limited by pain.

Unfortunately, diabetes is a risk factor for coronary artery disease, too. That is, diabetics are more likely to experience narrowing of the vital arteries in the heart that deliver blood and oxygen to the constantly moving heart muscle. My patient arrived in the emergency room one night—why do these crises always occur at night?—with crushing chest pain. Emergency evaluation by a cardiologist confirmed the obvious: his pain was angina, a precursor to a heart attack. Within hours, he had had surgery to bypass the narrowed area of his coronary artery, which could have caused a possibly fatal heart attack.

I was called to see him in the postoperative intensive care unit. The surgeon was proud of the work he had done, and rightfully so. His skill, like that of the cardiologist, had been vital in saving this man's life. But the patient was not so happy. He was experiencing excruciating pain. He felt as if someone had just stabbed a knife into his chest—as, indeed, had happened.

The surgeon was annoyed with the patient. He couldn't understand why twice the usual dose of morphine he prescribed for postoperative pain was inadequate for this patient. Why, the patient should be grateful that he had saved his life, and instead he was just griping about pain, and demanding more and more pain medicine!

In fact, even before he had come to the hospital, the patient's chronic methadone dose had been the equivalent of ten times the dose of morphine prescribed by the surgeon. That dose was fine for the chronic pain of the legs and flanks, but now he had acute pain too. I sat down by his bedside, and carefully injected syringe-full after syringe-full of morphine until the patient was comfortable. I wanted to use morphine rather than methadone to relieve the acute pain because it is easier to change the dose of morphine rapidly. That would give me more flexibility to match the dose of pain reliever to the patient's pain. After the initial injections of morphine relieved his pain, I calculated the equivalent dose to be given continuously to maintain that pain relief.

The tricky part was the subsequent dose adjustment. Since he was no longer taking methadone by mouth, the amount of that drug in his blood was slowly dropping. At the same time, the chest pain, so severe at first, was rapidly improving as he healed. There are no textbooks to guide the detailed adminis-tration of morphine in this setting, so I had to adjust the mor-phine dose regularly depending on his response to it. Of course, that is what should be done in any case. Even though he was opioid tolerant, the patient became drowsy during the next few days. That was a sign that his need for morphine was dropping as his acute pain was subsiding. I reduced the morphine dose rapidly, although not as rapidly as I had raised it. Within a week or two, his pain relief requirement was back to where it had been before admission.

CHAPTER 7

———————■———————

Treating Pain when Cancer Has Spread to Bones

Not long ago, and in a land not far away, cancer was so dread a disease that people were loath to even to mention its name. The disease was obliquely referred to as "the big C," or as "a growth." If the patient succumbed, the obituary would often read that death came after a "lengthy illness," in much the same way that death notices about HIV victims were worded in the early days of the AIDS epidemic. In some cases, cancer patients were even shunned by long-time friends as if the malady were somehow contagious.

Part of the fear, of course, arose from the fact that cancer was—and remains—a disease that is often fatal. But that is not the whole story. Heart disease caused death more frequently than cancer, and yet society never shuddered collectively in revulsion at the prospect of a heart attack. Then, too, cancer's potential to cause disfigurement may have been a factor in society's revulsion. Yet, osteoporosis can cause severe back deformity that is more disfiguring, but it never carried the emotional punch of cancer. So what distinguished cancer from other deadly or disfiguring diseases? We think that the primary cause of people's revulsion to cancer came from the fact that, in the past, dying from cancer could be a writhing, excruciating experience in which the only choice for the patient in severe pain was either agony or sedation.

That was yesterday. Today, cancer is one of the most publicized of diseases. Increasing cancer awareness is a major goal of public health education efforts. Famous movie stars and politicians—the very kinds of celebrities who would have once moved heaven and

105

earth to keep their cancers secret—now routinely appear on television and the radio to discuss their struggles. Why the change? Part of it has to do, no doubt, with the increased openness of contemporary times. But we also believe that the new openness in discussing cancer comes, at least in part, from the encouraging success achieved by modern medicine in controlling cancer pain. Regardless of whether that is so, we hope that this book, and especially this chapter, will make a significant contribution to knocking cancer off its pedestal of terror.

First and foremost, we wish to emphasize that *virtually all cancer pain can be substantially alleviated or even eliminated.* We have already discussed much of how this is accomplished in the chapters on opioids (Chapter 4) and the treatment of chronic pain (Chapter 5). Still, a few points are worth reemphasizing:

- When there is no anti-cancer treatment that will help the patient, much can still be done to treat the cancer-related pain. Most patients—some estimate as many as 90 percent—can find relief with the oral medicine discussed earlier in the chapter on the management of chronic pain. Almost all of the rest can find relief via other forms of care, many of which will be described later in this chapter.

- As with other chronic pain, cancer pain should be treated ATC (around the clock), not just prn (as needed). If a doctor prescribes, or a patient takes pain control medicine for cancer "as needed," it is almost a guarantee that the patient will have the miserable roller coaster ride of pain-pill-relief, pain-pill-relief. He learns to dread the passing hours, since they will bring with him a reminder of the cancer, and a return of the dreaded pain.

- The mainstay of cancer pain treatment is opioids. These may be taken orally, or worn as a patch that delivers the medicine

106

round the clock. Which drug is taken—there are several—is less important than that it be taken ATC and in proper dose.

- If the cancer worsens, the dose requirement may rise. Similarly, if the cancer improves, due to, for example, chemotherapy or radiation therapy, the dose requirement may drop. It is completely irrelevant how many milligrams of a drug the patient takes per day. It is more than relevant—indeed it is *vital* to the whole purpose of the enterprise—that pain be completely controlled. If the doctor says, "I'm worried about how much medicine you're taking," the patient should reply, "That's funny. I'm worried about how much pain I would be having if I weren't taking it."

In many cases, treating pain caused by cancer may be easier than treating many other forms of chronic pain. However, cancer does present some unique issues in pain control that require discussion in their own chapter. Most of these have to do with some cancers' propensity to spread to the bones

Years ago, when standard cancer therapy was less effective and more toxic than it is today, treatments were often derided as "cut it, burn it, or poison it" medicine, referring to surgery, radiation therapy, and chemotherapy. Today, we don't often hear these treatments so negatively described because their benefit, even though sometimes tragically limited, is widely recognized. What is not widely recognized, however, is that these treatments can sometimes be useful in treating not merely the cancer, but also its pain.

This is particularly true in cases where cancer has spread—in a process known as metastasizing—to the bones. Mostly, these are bones in the center of the body, such as the ribs, vertebrae, and pelvis. Metastases to the long bones, such as the femur in the thigh and the humerus in the upper arm, are somewhat less common, but still occur often enough to be a particular concern.

Metastases to the long bones can be doubly problematic. First, of course, they hurt, and they hurt more during weight bearing. Secondly, some tumors can actually erode the bone, eating right through it to cause a fracture.

 ___*From the Doctor's Journal:*___

From time to time I have seen patients whose first recognized symptom of cancer was a fracture due to a bone metastasis, that is, spread of cancer to the bone. In these cases, the tumor steadily erodes through the bone. The patient may have pain, but, in these cases I'm recalling now, the pain was not severe enough to bring the patient to the doctor. After the tumor has eroded through the majority of the cortex (thick outer part) of the bone, it takes trivial force to complete the fracture. This may be compared to a tree that has been sawed almost completely through. A little girl pushing on the tree may then be able to bring it crashing down to the forest floor.

The final event in the progression of a bone metastasis, like the straw that breaks a camel's back, is usually well remembered by the patient. I, too, remember them. One elderly patient with lung cancer that had spread to her humerus (upper arm) told me that she had had an annoying ache in her arm for several weeks. Then, one day, she opened the refrigerator door. As she pulled on the door, she felt a sudden snapping sensation in her arm, followed by severe pain there. She had just broken her arm. Another patient with metastatic lung cancer told me how he had had some aching in his thigh until he stepped down from a curb, and then suddenly felt a sharp pain at the old achy site. He had just completed the fracture of his femur. These fractures, called pathological fractures, are usually easy to distinguish from traumatic fractures, those that occur due to injuries. In pathological fractures, the force involved, as in these episodes at the refrigerator and the curb, are ordinary.

■

Detecting Cancer in the Bones

Fortunately, early intervention can prevent this major complication and the pain that comes with it. The first step in preventing severe pain from bone metastases is to detect them before fracturing occurs. This can be done by using a medical process known as bone scanning, an imaging technique that is particularly sensitive in detecting bone metastases. First, a tiny dose of a radioactive material is injected in the vein. This harmless amount of radioactive material (usually called a "radionuclide") circulates through the body and is removed from the blood stream by cells in the bones. Bone cells near cancer metastases are particularly active at absorbing the radionuclide. Since the radionuclide emits a low amount of x-rays, bone tumor sites will emit more x-rays than normal bone. Normal bone, in turn, emits more x-rays than does the rest of the body.

The next step is to pass a Geiger counter attached to a camera in front and in back of the patient's body, thereby making a picture reflecting the variable distribution of the radioactivity. Sites that emit excessive radioactivity are called "hot spots" by doctors, although their temperature is really no different from that of the rest of the body. The bone scan is so sensitive that it routinely reveals bone metastases about which the patient is not yet aware. (Other diseases besides cancer may cause an abnormal bone scan, but radiologists can usually easily distinguish these from cases of bone metastases.)

Finally, if the bone scan shows hot spots in the femur or humerus, the doctor can monitor the activity of the cancer at that site. Curiously, the best way to monitor this is not by repeating the bone scan, but by monitoring the patient's symptoms and x-rays. Bone scans are too sensitive for monitoring. But the x-ray, unlike the bone scan, reflects the structural integrity of the bone, that is, the x-ray will reflect whether and how far the bone has eroded. Thus, if the bone scan is abnormal but the x-ray is normal, the patient may have cancer in the bone, but it is not likely to fracture the bone soon. On the other hand, if the x-ray shows that the tumor has eroded through the majority of the bone, the doctors can predict that this is a site of likely fracture.

Surgery

Different bones require different treatment if they are in danger of breaking. In this regard, the femur may be the easiest to treat through a remarkably safe and effective surgical procedure. The orthopedic surgeon makes an incision at the hip, and inserts a metal rod down the shaft of the bone through the damaged area into the normal bone beyond it. The metal rod is held in place by a chemical with the almost impossible-to-pronounce name "methylmethacrylate." It is essentially akin to Super Glue. This operation immediately strengthens the bone, allowing the patient to safely bear weight on it even hours after the operation. The total time in the hospital may be just a few days. This kind of surgery does not cure the cancer; it may not even prolong life. But it does relieve pain and prevent the ongoing disability that a fracture would cause, adding immeasurably to the patient's quality of life.

There is no analogous operation that can be performed on ribs, and the surgery needed for metastases in the arm bone (humerus) is a bit more complicated. Metastases to the backbone (vertebra) are usually best managed by radiation therapy and analgesics, but there are cases there, too, in which surgery can be quite useful.

110

From the Doctor's Journal:

I remember a case in which I chose the wrong therapy for a patient, but the outcome was happy nonetheless. I mention this case, despite the fact that it reflects my mistake, because it is important to emphasize that no one doctor knows it all.

I was treating a middle-aged man for metastatic kidney cancer. It had spread to the soft tissue next to one of his vertebrae, and he still had pain there after radiation therapy. Drug therapy of the cancer itself had little to offer. I explained that the drug is fairly toxic and that a majority of the patients treated with it have no benefit. Still, I wanted to inform the patient of its availability, since he might look on a 15 percent likelihood of benefit differently than I did. He knew that the drug would not cure the cancer, and he elected wisely, I think, not to receive it.

The pain was a different matter. I thought that the best management for the pain would be oral analgesics. He wanted to get a second opinion at a regional referral center, so I quickly arranged for it. I'm glad he did want to get that opinion, because the other doctor's advice was better than mine. He saw a specialist in vertebral surgery, who recommended that this isolated metastasis be removed and the vertebra rebuilt and stabilized with artificial material. The patient got through the surgery fine, and now has much better pain control. He still needs to take some oral analgesics, but his dose is lower and the benefit is greater than it would have been if he had not had the surgery. We both benefited from his seeing the surgeon. As my wife often reminds me, "M.D." does not stand for "Medical Deity"; nobody knows it all.

Radiation

The best bet for cancer patients with bone involvement is to prevent the metastasis from progressing to the point where surgery is necessary. Fortunately, there is often much that can be done in this regard. Although radiation therapy will not prevent a fracture in a bone on the verge of breaking, it can both reduce pain and reduce the risk of fracture if it is used before the crisis arises.

Radiation usually involves a number of visits to the radiation therapy center. The patient lies down on a table, and a beam of x-rays is aimed at the site of the bone tumor. The patient does not feel the x-rays any more than he would feel a beam of light from a flashlight. This therapy takes only a few minutes a day. Typically it can be completed in a few weeks, and there are some circumstances in which the whole dose can be given in a single session.

The radiation therapy often causes a transient sunburn-like effect at the site of its application. Nausea may occur, but it is less frequent when bone metastases are irradiated than when other cancer sites are exposed to radiation. Fatigue is a common side effect. Since normal marrow inevitably is included in the irradiation field, there may be some drop in the number of circulating blood cells. (Blood is manufactured in the marrow.) This can lead to symptomatic anemia, and, less commonly, an increased risk of infection or bleeding.

A new way of irradiating painful bone metastases has recently become available that adds to the ability of radiology to treat bone cancer. This involves the use of *therapeutic* radionuclides, that is, the injection of radioactive material that not only detects bone cancer spots, but also treats them. You will recall from a few pages ago that when a bone scan is done, the radioactive material is picked up by the bone tumor sites. From there it emits a harmless dose of radiation. In bone scanning, the radionuclide emits the kind of radiation with which we're most familiar—x-rays (also called gamma rays). This form of radiation is so energetic that it goes all the way through the soft tissue

112

surrounding the bone to arrive at the Geiger counter camera. (That is how it is possible to make a picture of the inside of the body with x-rays.)

But what if there were a form of irradiation that traveled only a few millimeters before it was absorbed and gave off its energy? This radiation could be used as a treatment from the inside in much the same way as external radiation therapy works from the outside, but without being nearly as harmful to healthy tissues. We now have such an injectable treatment available. It is called beta irradiation.

Beta irradiation works like a bone scan, only better. First, the doctor injects the beta radionuclide. Just as in the case of the x-ray radionuclide, its beta ray cousin is taken up preferentially at sites of bone metastases. The radiation it emits does not travel as far as does the x-ray energy of bone scans. Instead, it is absorbed by the cancer cells near the bone cells that have picked up the radionuclide, killing a goodly number of them. The result is a decrease in the number of the cancer cells and a consequent improvement in the bone pain.

Two therapeutic radionuclides are now available. One is strontium-89, whose trade name is Metastron®. The other is samarium-153, whose trade name is Quadramet®. From the patient's point of view, there are only minor differences between the two of them.

Unlike external beam irradiation, therapeutic radionuclides, administered in a single injection, can simultaneously treat all the sites of bone metastases. Moreover, that one injection can be combined with external beam irradiation. Indeed, in 1993, Dr. A.T. Porter and co-workers published a study in *The International Journal of Radiation Oncology, Biology, and Physics* describing the care of men whose prostate cancers had spread to the bone. The study compared the use of external irradiation alone to external irradiation in combination with a therapeutic radionuclide. That study found that the patients who received the combination therapy had fewer symptoms of painful bone metastases during the rest of their lives compared with men who re-

113

ceived only the external beam irradiation. The study only applies formally to prostate cancer that has spread to the bone, but its conclusions are a hopeful sign for other types of cancer with bone involvement.

There is a downside to therapeutic radionuclides. The disadvantage is that they suppress marrow function more than does external beam irradiation of a single site. When the marrow is suppressed, it is less able to make red cells, white cells, and platelets. Stating that a patient has insufficient red cells is just another way of describing anemia. That causes fatigue and breathlessness. The job of the white cells is to fight infection, so, when the number circulating in the blood stream is quite low, the risk of serious infection rises sharply. The job of the platelets is to help the blood clot normally. So a patient with a low platelet count is at risk of bleeding and bruising. The key in using both external irradiation and therapeutic radionuclide is to choose a dose that maximizes the harm to the cancer while minimizing the harm to the normal marrow.

There is another disadvantage that comes along with marrow suppression. Marrow suppression from radiation therapy (external or by therapeutic radionuclide) may bar the use of chemotherapy later in the course of the patient's illness, since chemotherapy can also be toxic to the bone marrow. Another disadvantage, of course, is that therapeutic radionuclides are useful only in cases of bone metastases, and have no role in the management of cancer that has spread to soft tissues, such as lung or lymph nodes.

Another problem surrounding this beneficial type of treatment for bone cancers has nothing to do with biology. Therapeutic radionuclides are sometimes called an orphan therapy because they may be difficult to obtain. Part of the problem involves logistics. Therapeutic radionuclide therapy requires special equipment to safely store the radioactive material used in this kind of treatment. Thus, it is not usually available in the private offices of medical oncologists or radiation oncologists. Instead, patients must go to a radiologist in the nuclear medicine department of a hospital for the care. Since these departments are very busy places, scheduling can be a problem.

A more significant issue in obtaining this kind of therapy is that nuclear medicine doctors are usually "out of the loop" in treating cancer, since their primary responsibility is reading diagnostic images. And since medical and radiation oncologists usually don't deal with therapeutic radionuclides on a daily basis, it is easy to forget about the availability and effectiveness of this unique therapy. Making matters worse, radiation oncologists often fail to refer patients for this therapy when it might offer some benefit. This is not because, as some cynics have argued, that they earn no income when the patient receives therapeutic radionuclides rather than external beam irradiation. Rather, it is because people honestly have more confidence in and give more thought to therapies with which they are personally familiar and which they themselves are experienced in administering. This means you should be prepared to bring up the subject yourself. *If you or a loved one has bone metastases, be sure to ask whether radionuclide therapy would be a beneficial approach in your particular case.*

Medicine

There is an even less toxic therapy that is remarkably effective in diminishing or preventing bone pain from metastatic cancer. That is pamidronate (trade name Aredia®). Pamidronate does not kill cancer cells. Rather, it blocks the ability of the cancer cells in the bone to eat away at the bone. You see, cancer cells do not directly eat away at bones. Rather, they wreak their destruction by stimulating normal cells in the bone to remove minerals. This breaking down of the bone's mineral content is a perfectly natural process, as is the building up of bone that goes on at the same time. Ordinarily, the two factors are well balanced so that the mineral content of the bone stays stable over time.

Some diseases or injuries cause an imbalance between these two functions. Osteoporosis, for example, is the consequence of bone breakdown slightly exceeding bone buildup over many years. During repair of a fracture, on the other hand, the bone buildup exceeds the breakdown, a healthy response to the injury.

Pamidronate works by blocking the activity of the cells that break down bones. It has been proven to reduce bone pain and fractures in metastatic breast cancer that has spread to the bone, and in myeloma, where the bone is the original cancer site. It is likely that the same benefit exists in other cancers that eat away at bone.

The drug is ordinarily administered intravenously once a month. It may cause a low-grade fever the first time it is given, but major side effects with this drug are rare. It does not suppress marrow function, and it does not cause hair loss.

 From the Doctor's Journal:

The availability of pamidronate has made myeloma virtually a different disease in my practice from what it was when I first became an oncologist. (Myeloma is often called "bone cancer," although more accurately it should be called "bone marrow cancer." It is a malignancy that arises in the marrow, and then spreads out to erode the bones.) In the bad old days, I could expect my myeloma patients to suffer one bone fracture after another. The fractures were very painful, of course, and seldom healed completely. This made myeloma perhaps the most feared cancer.

I remember a man named Frank. He was about 65 years-old when I was treating him for myeloma in the pre-pamidronate days. Frank had the custom of wearing his trousers rather high above the waist. That had nothing to do with his myeloma; it was just his fashion. But I noticed that over the months and then the few years that I treated Frank, he began to wear his trousers rolled up at the cuff. Toward the end of his life, his trousers were rolled up to a considerable degree.

The reason for this was that Frank suffered from progressive compression fractures of the lumbar vertebrae. The best way to understand this is to imagine a stack of empty cardboard boxes.

116

If too much weight is put on them, they'll scrunch down, each one being compressed from its former size. So it is with compression fractures of the spine. The vertebrae do not break in pieces. Rather, they scrunch down within themselves, with the bony cortex ("crust") of the bone being pushed into the soft marrow within the bone. The rolled up trousers told the whole story. He was losing height from progressive compression fractures of the spine, and the pain from the disease prevented him from going to a store to buy new trousers.

Today, patients with myeloma seldom have the progressive debility and pain of numerous bone fractures, thanks to pamidronate. One of my current patients is a man in his mid-fifties whose myeloma was treated (but not, unfortunately, cured) with a bone marrow transplant. His only therapy now is monthly infusions of pamidronate. Despite his disease, he works full time as a manufacturer's representative. His hobby? He is a referee for college and high school basketball! That is an example of the difference that pamidronate has made in the lives of my patients. In the near future, I expect drugs similar but better than pamidronate to be available to prevent bone pain and fractures

Drug Therapy As Pain Control

A discussion of the management of cancer pain would be incomplete without a mention of drug therapy. Cancer drug therapy may be given intravenously, orally, or by other routes. The term is meant to exclude other forms of cancer therapy, such as surgery, irradiation, physical therapy, etc.

Broadly speaking, drug therapy of cancer may be divided into different subtypes. These are cytotoxic (cell-killing) chemotherapy, immunotherapy, and hormone therapy. In the future there will probably be other kinds of drug therapy, involving insertion of new genes into normal or cancer cells, or blocking the function of deranged genes within the cancer cell. But that will be the topic for another book.

Cytotoxic chemotherapy uses the kinds of drugs most people think of when they think of chemotherapy. Most of them work by disrupting the normal function of DNA in cells. This either directly kills the cancer cells or induces them to activate a self-destruct mechanism, called apoptosis. Unfortunately, most of these drugs also damage normal cells. This leads to the well-known toxic side effects of the drugs. The usefulness of chemotherapy comes from the fact that most normal tissues recover from the toxic effect of chemotherapy faster than do the malignant cells.

The difficult job of the oncologist is to balance the risks and benefits of these drugs. That is, the oncologist must prescribe enough chemotherapy to significantly harm the cancer but not so much as to destroy too many normal cells. This is no easy task. Since virtually no single dose of chemotherapy will completely rid the entire body of cancer, multiple dosing is usually necessary. But any cells that survive the first barrage of chemotherapy may give rise to daughter cells that are also resistant to the drugs used. Thus, after a few cycles of chemotherapy all the remaining malignant cells in the body are either intrinsically resistant or are the descendants of multiple "ancestor cells" previously resistant to the drugs.

An analogy can be made to mosquitoes and insecticide. The first spraying of a field of mosquitoes will kill 90 percent of the insects. The next season there may be fewer mosquitoes, but all of the mosquitoes are children of insects that were resistant to the insecticide. If the field is sprayed again, perhaps 50 percent of the insects will be killed. By the next summer the population of mosquitoes will be greater, and now all the insects will be descended from both parents and grandparents who were resistant to the insecticide. Spraying the field now may result in the killing of only 10 percent of the mosquitoes. This repeated spraying has selected a strain of insects that are resistant to the insecticide.

Similarly, the initial chemotherapy of cancer may significantly shrink the tumor. The next cycle of chemotherapy may shrink the tumor a little further, but eventually subsequent cycles may have no impact at all. After a few cycles of chemotherapy, the tumor is completely resistant to the therapy that had once been dramatically effective.

Unlike cancer cells, normal cells do not ordinarily change the pattern of their DNA from one generation of cells to the next. When, for example, a normal ancestor liver cell divides, it will create a liver cell virtually identical to the one it will make tomorrow and the day after. That is both good news and bad news. It is good news because changing DNA from one generation to the next is one mechanism by which cancer arises. It is bad news since the normal cells cannot acquire a resistance to the effects of chemotherapy, as do the malignant cells. Thus, although the benefit of chemotherapy usually diminishes with repeat exposure to the drug, the side effects of chemotherapy usually do not.

Chemotherapy may be used to treat cancer in two different situations. One is that in which there is a reasonable chance of curing the patient with chemotherapy, meaning you kill all the cancer cells so that resistant ones do not grow to form new tumors. The other is when cure is impossible or highly unlikely, and the goal of the chemotherapy is to reduce symptoms and/or prolong life.

When chemotherapy is given with curative intent, then we are not as deterred by side effects. If the chemotherapy causes hair loss, fatigue, nausea, or pain, most people feel that these temporary side effects are a reasonable, if not small, price to pay to be cured of a potentially fatal illness. There are several cancers now in which cure is commonly achieved and whose chemotherapy most people consider well worth the benefit. These include testicular cancer, Hodgkin's disease, some non-Hodgkin's lymphomas, some forms of leukemia, etc.

119

The calculation is more difficult, however, when the chemo-therapy will surely not be curative. Then, the doctor and patient have to weigh and consider how much side effect is worth how much pro-longation of life or reduction in cancer symptoms.

There are a number of cancers in which the benefit is not cure, but prolongation of life by many months or years. These include ova-rian cancer, metastatic breast cancer, and small cell lung cancer. The patient is usually sick when starting treatment and feels better as a result. Easy decision.

In other cases the chemotherapy is not proven to prolong life, so its only purpose is to diminish cancer-related symptoms, including pain. Here, the doctor must choose relatively mild therapies, since harsh therapies might cause symptoms worse than those being treated. Patients with metastatic prostate cancer or pancreatic cancer, for ex-ample, may not have life prolonged by chemotherapy, but may enjoy symptom reduction.

One of the cancer symptoms that may be reduced by chemotherapy is pain. A good example is the treatment of prostate cancer no longer responsive to hormone therapy. While chemotherapy has not been proven to prolong survival, it does often improve some symptoms. Whether that improvement can be achieved as well with other thera-pies, or whether in the particular case the adverse effects exceed the benefit, must be decided on a case-by-case basis.

The point is that chemotherapy, too, has a potential role in the treatment of cancer pain and should at least be considered when determining the best approach to pain relief. However, the goal of the therapy—whether it is curative, life prolonging, or symptom reducing—should be discussed by the patient and doctor before the therapy begins in order to avoid any misunderstanding. Doc-tors have a duty to inform the patient of the treatment options, to be very clear as to recommendations, and then to accept the deci-sion of the patient.

Pain Control at the End of Life

A few further words need to be said about pain control in the final days and hours of life. Many patients needlessly fear that they must choose between alertness and pain relief in this critical time. In fact, that is not so. Many people, of course, become less alert in the days before death and spend much time asleep or seemingly confused. This is often simply part of the dying process, and it is not worsened nor helped by the pain medicine. What pain control can definitely improve, however, is the comfort that the dying person has as life ebbs away.

Some family members are reluctant to continue opioids when the patient is dying of cancer because they are fearful that the drug will inadvertently shorten life. They can be reassured on several levels. First, there is no evidence at all that continuing opioids in this circumstance shortens life. We do know, however, that continuing opioid medication as the patient is dying prevents the re-emergence of pain or the precipitation of an uncomfortable withdrawal syndrome. Morphine given to the dying is not some sleight of hand by which doctors secretly euthanize their patients. It is pain relief given to maximize the quality of the final precious days of life. (We will go into more details about pain control at the end of life in the next chapter.)

CHAPTER 8

Hospice:
The True Death with Dignity

Unpleasant as it may be to contemplate, there comes a time in each of our lives when we must, as Shakespeare so artfully put it, "shuffle off this mortal coil." While it is certainly true that, ultimately, death cannot be prevented, it can often be significantly delayed with the miracles of modern medicine. But what happens when treatment no longer holds out any realistic chance of cure or significant life extension? That is the time to consider a unique form of medical care, one that has been specifically designed to assist dying people and their families through this difficult time. This form of care has a name: hospice.

Hospice is a term that identifies special forms of medical treatment and care for dying people. Most people know that hospice places special emphasis on pain control, particularly on using morphine and other opioids as aggressively as is necessary to keep the patient comfortable. But hospice is so much more than that. It involves what medical types call a "multidisciplinary approach" to patient care. That is, it involves medical treatment, nursing care, social services, spiritual and pastoral intervention for those who want it, community involvement through volunteers, and assistance for families, among other services.

Too many people in this country believe that hospice is about hopelessness. To the contrary. Hospice is actually about hope. It is about compassion, inclusion, and a community's care and love for people whose lives are ending. Those who are still relatively healthy and have not had a loved one cared for by hospice may find this optimistic assessment difficult to understand. But, since hospice came into vogue a little more than 30 years ago, hundreds of thousands of patients and families have benefited from its unique loving care. Strange as it may sound, the dying are living proof of hospice's uplifting approach to the needs of the terminally ill. They stand witness to the fact that, even at the time of greatest stress and sorrow, there may yet be hope. And they demonstrate the truth of the words of Rabbi Harold Kushner, author of *When Bad Things Happen To Good People* (Schocken Books [1981], 2001), who wrote, "There may not be a chance for a cure, but there is always an opportunity for healing."

Bringing Humanity Back into Dying

Hospice represents a return to the wisdom of community care, arguably the finest achievement in treating patients before the modern era of medicine. Somehow western medicine, in its understandably heady delight over its technological achievements, lost sight of the human element. It acted as if we were not mortal, as if death were not our certain and ultimate fate, no matter how successful medicine became.

Medicine was once as much an art as a science, and dying was as much a part of the daily lives of the community as was birth. In those days, dying people were not shunned and isolated as they often are today. They weren't looked upon as if they were somehow a different form of life. When dying people could no longer go out into the community, the community came to them. Families came together to share the responsibilities of care; friends and associates visited often and picked up the slack when necessary; children played noisily in the next room. As a result, dying people did not feel ostracized from life, or that they were somehow "a burden." In short, death was simply a part of life, and caring for each other was the norm, merely a part of our human obligation to each other. An unspoken social contract prevailed: today I care for a loved one, and, when my time comes, others will care me for.

With the advent of technological medicine, dying lost much of its humanity. People stopped dying at home, and all too many ended their days hooked up to machines in hospitals as doctors struggled mightily to maintain life one more week, one more day, one more hour. Of course, extending life has always been a primary purpose of medicine. The problem came when life extension became an obsession—the end all and be all of patient treatment—to the exclusion of dignity and patient autonomy. Although the actual number of such cases was a small percentage of the total deaths, the way that some doctors refused to stop unwanted medical treatment outraged the public. Too often, it seemed that doctors were forcing patients to remain alive under intensive care—the infamous hooking up to machines against their will—when all the patients wanted was to be allowed to die at home, in their own beds, surrounded by loved ones and friends, in comfort, dignity, and peace.

Many doctors felt as frustrated by this outcome as did the patients and families. In addition, the doctors often feared that they would be sued if they were seen to "just let the patient die" without an effort to prevent the death. Equally influential was the culture in which the doctors worked. Any patient's death was viewed as a defeat. Like the patients and families, many doctors felt that somehow the system had gone astray, but they had no good model of how to correct it.

Eventually people rebelled at what they saw as medical despotism. This rebellion took both a negative and a positive form. Some used the opportunity to promote the false compassion of assisted suicide and euthanasia as the answer to medicalized dying. But, long before anyone had ever heard of Jack Kevorkian, the true path to "death with dignity" was already being blazed by a wonderful British physician named Cicely Saunders (now, Dame Saunders). Between the years 1946 and 1967, this little English giant of compassionate care developed the concept of the modern hospice.

While caring for a dying holocaust survivor in the immediate aftermath of World War II, Saunders had a compelling insight about how to better care for dying people. At the time, Saunders was a nurse and medical social worker. She realized that dying people were receiving inadequate care, often dying in pain with the family virtually ignored by the medical system. So, she went to medical school at the age of 33, and, upon becoming a physician, chose to specialize in the care of dying people, an unheard of concept at the time.

In a December 1998 interview with this book's co-author, Wesley J. Smith, Dame Saunders talked about the early development of the hospice concept. "I coined the term 'total pain' to describe how dying people experience physical, psychological, social, and spiritual pain. The patient needs care in all of these areas. So I started studying how to accomplish this, and also spent a great deal of time raising money, so that I could open a hospice that treated the whole patient."

Saunders' dream came true in 1967 with the opening of St. Christopher's Hospice in a suburb of London. As happy as Saunders was at having a hospice facility where dying people could come for care, she knew that most people preferred to die in their own homes. As a consequence, Saunders developed hospice as an in-home form of care, beginning in 1969. Hospice was received so enthusiastically by both doctors and patients that Dame Saunders exported the concept to the United States in 1971. Today, although retired from the active practice of medicine, Saunders still promotes hospice throughout the world. She spends her days writing and meeting the many dignitaries, physicians, and hospice workers who make their way to her second floor office at St. Christopher's. What is Dame Saunders' current project? To bring the comfort and dignity of hospice to the undeveloped world.

So what exactly is hospice care? Hospice has been described as both a philosophy and a treatment. It is care, primarily based in the home, intended to maximize the quality and dignity of a person's life as death approaches, usually without treating the underlying disease that is leading to death. This is because the underlying disease is either fundamentally untreatable, has reached a phase in which it is resistant to treatment, or the patient has decided to allow nature to take its course. As we will describe below, hospice care is best known for its pain and symptom control, but it also pays significant attention to the social and spiritual needs of the patient and the family.

In the United States, the majority of hospice patients are seniors, so their hospice care is paid for by Medicare and, to varying degrees, by most health insurance policies. There is a catch, though. Unlike in England, which permits people in hospice to also receive potentially curative treatment, people who are eligible for Medicare may elect to receive either hospice care *or* disease-oriented treatment of their terminal illness. According to Dame Saunders, this either/or approach is one reason why hospice is so underutilized in the United States. Thus, patients with newly diagnosed metastatic breast cancer should usually not choose hospice care, since treatment of metastatic breast cancer can usually add years and quality to a person's life. Similarly, congestive heart failure and emphysema in their early stages clearly benefit from medical management.

But many diseases progress despite treatment. When the doctor says that attempts at curative treatment are not likely to hold death at bay, that is the not the time to give up on the medical system.

Some doctors even say, "There is nothing more I can do."

Wrong! There *never* comes a time when nothing more can be done for the patient. When curative or life-prolonging treatments are not longer available, or are too difficult for the patient, the time has come to think of switching to a hospice approach. However, the patient or family may have to bring up the subject, because too many doctors are reluctant to speak plainly to their patients about terminal diagnoses.

126

How Hospice Works

Many people fall into despair as their death approaches because they are under the misunderstanding that, in their final weeks and months of life, they must choose between miserable pain on the one hand, and being sedated to the point of stupor on the other. Fortunately, as described in Chapter 5, that is not at all the case. With proper hospice care, the final stage of life can be lived in peace, comfort, and dignity. Indeed, that is the goal of this compassionate form of care. Toward this end, hospice care provides patients with several important and overlapping services. These are:

- **Pain Control** – Ensuring a life free of degrading pain is Job One in hospice. Most often, this involves the aggressive use of pain-controlling medications such as morphine, which, you will remember, can be delivered in increasing doses if the pain caused by the illness increases. It is not unusual for an advanced stage cancer patient to receive high doses of morphine. Happily for the patient, who would otherwise be in agony, the morphine does not end life; it just ends intolerable pain. If necessary, hospice nurses will visit patients daily to ensure that their pain is under control. Most hospices have nurses on call around the clock 365 days a year, in the event of a pain emergency.

- **Symptom Management** – Hospice is also deeply concerned with controlling distressing physical symptoms other than pain that may be associated with dying. This form of care may include medication to treat nausea, depression, severe itching, breathlessness, or constipation. In fact, there is no symptom of terminal illness whose treatment is not a legitimate target of hospice care.

- **Personal Service Workers** – Hospice also provides important personal services for the patient, care that means so much at this time of life. These include rubbing cream on dry skin, changing dressings, and similar assistance of a personal nature. In this regard, most hospices have what is called a bath team. Many people who are terminally ill are too weak to bathe themselves, and often family members are also unable to bathe them. The hospice bath team comes into the home and bathes the patient. That may involve assisting the patient into and out of the tub or shower, or, if necessary, bathing the patient in bed. The team's skill in facilitating the bath in safety, despite the patient's weakness, helps maintain the patient in the dignity of cleanliness. No one has to die in pain; no one has to die dirty. The look in a patient's eyes at being so lovingly cared for is mute testimony to the importance of this compassionate service.

- **Social Work** – Social workers assess the patient and the family situation to help access government and insurance benefits to which they may be entitled, and to help coordinate the totality of care. The importance of the social worker is often underestimated. At the end of life, the last thing the sick person or family members need is a bureaucratic hassle. Yet the fact is that there are often a lot of nonmedical decisions to be made. Funeral plans must be considered. Getting relatives released from job responsibilities under the Family Medical Leave Act often requires some jumping through paperwork hoops. While social workers cannot replace competent lawyers, they are knowledgeable about some of the legal decisions—concerning wills, adoptions, etc.—that may be necessary at this time. When patients cannot afford a lawyer, social workers are often able to guide them to sources of free or inexpensive legal counsel. Sometimes the social worker will find a home for a dear pet that will outlive the patient. This, too, can be a great source of comfort.

The death of a patient does not magically transform a family that has been living in friction into a modern day Ozzie and Harriet Nelson clan. The reality is that the interpersonal frictions that pre-existed the illness are magnified, not erased, by the stress of a terminal illness. Social workers do not necessarily eliminate the frictions, but they are skilled at helping family members work as a team to focus on the job of caring for the dying relative; their interpersonal squabbles can be put on hold.

- **Psychological/Emotional Support** – Psychologists, therapists, and bereavement counselors provide valuable grief counseling and emotional support. And not just to the patient. The family is also eligible for these services both before and after the death.

 From the Desk of WJS:

When my father was dying, I had to face not only my own grief, but my mother's as well. As an only child, the duty of caring for my parents' differing problems, caused by my father's impending death, fell exclusively on my shoulders. Knowing that I needed professional help so that I could help my parents, I obtained grief counseling through hospice. It made all the difference. My father died in hospice, peacefully and with dignity. And because of grief counseling, I was able to help not only my father, but also my mother (and myself) through a very difficult time.

- **Chaplain Services** – The role of hospice chaplains is some-times misunderstood. They are often erroneously thought to be replacements for the patients' own clergy members, or as individuals who seek to promote their own religions. That is not at all the case. Most dying patients (like most healthy people) have spiritual needs, and they are often prominently in mind as death approaches. The chaplain's role is to help the patient achieve spiritual comfort within the framework of the patient's (as opposed to the chaplain's) own religions sys-tem. A Christian chaplain can bring as much comfort to a Jewish patient as can a Jewish chaplain to a Christian one. The chaplain sits at the bedside, talking or praying with the dying patient, if that is what the patient or the family desires. If the patient is too weak to talk, the chaplain may just read quietly to the patient. Sometimes the chaplain is simply there. This has been referred to as the ministry of presence.

- **Respite Care** – While some dying people enter in-patient hospice facilities, the vast majority of hospice treatment oc-curs in the patient's home with the aid of family members and friends. Because caregiving is an emotionally intense and sometimes exhausting experience, it often helps the family to "get away" for some time of respite. Thus, hospice will pay for caregiving in respite centers for brief periods of time to permit families to recharge their physical and emotional batteries.

- **Volunteers** – Many hospices maintain a group of volunteers, people from the community who are trained by the hospice to perform invaluable services that fall outside of "profes-sional" duties. Volunteers help patients and their families in so many ways. One important task often undertaken by vol-unteers is simply giving the primary caregiver a break from daily duties. The volunteer will sit with the patient while the

130

primary caregiver goes shopping, gets a haircut or perm, or just gets away for some badly needed time alone. Volunteers may help in a variety of other ways as well. For example, the volunteer might pick up some groceries for the family, or watch young children while the parents are visiting the doctor. Others might do some light tidying of the house or preparation of some meals. Hospice volunteers also alert the hospice team if something seems amiss. For example, it is not rare for patients to disclose problems to the volunteer that they keep from the nurse, since some people find it easier to be open with "real people" than they do with health care professionals. In short, the hospice volunteer personifies the hospice philosophy of keeping the dying within the human community, including them in the world of the living rather than ignoring them as if they were already dead.

 ## *From the Desk of WJS:*

As I lecture around the country, appear on talk radio, and otherwise interact with the public about the issue of biomedical ethics, audience members often ask me what they can do to make life better for dying people. I always have an immediate answer: "Become a hospice volunteer."

Too often, people who are nearing the end of their lives find themselves feeling abandoned and isolated. One of the most depressing causes of this sense of isolation is the loss of contact with friends and loved ones. It isn't as if the friends or relatives of the dying person no longer care. They do, deeply. But in our death-denying culture, many find it difficult to visit with a person whom they expect to die in a short period of time. We fear becoming emotionally upset or worry that we will somehow say the "wrong thing" and, thus, "make matters worse."

This is the wrong strategy. It often leaves patients feeling as if they are no longer worthy of love or concern, that they might as well be dead already. As one of the patients with whom I served as a hospice volunteer put it glumly, "First my friends stopped visiting me. Then my friends stopped calling me. Then they stopped calling my wife. Soon, I felt as if I were a token presence in the world." Hospice volunteers serve many roles, but their most important role may be as a living, breathing demonstration to dying patients that they remain valued as people and are still part of their community.

Serving as a hospice volunteer is a two-way street. Being a hospice volunteer is one of life's most rewarding and interesting experiences. I know that the people I have met, and the times I have shared with my hospice patients have changed my life. There was Ernie, an elderly Italian man diagnosed with terminal congestive heart failure. When I first met Ernie, he tearfully told me that he just wanted to die because he felt as if he was nothing but a burden. But during what were expected to be his final weeks, his family and friends convinced him that he remained valued and loved. I watched a wonderful and paradoxical transformation: Ernie began living again even as he prepared to die. Much to everyone's surprise, and to *his* most of all, Ernie did not die. His health improved to the point that he no longer needed hospice care. The last time I saw him, he played an Italian song for me on his mandolin.

Then there was the elderly woman—a flapper in the 1920s and a part of the New York music scene throughout the pre-War years— whom I took home from the doctor's office one day. What stories she told of the shows, the fun, the parties with George Gershwin playing his new tunes on the piano. After I helped her into her easy chair at her home, she asked me to help her out of her dress and into a robe. Then she asked me to get her nightgown out of the drawer so she could put it on after I left. She was wearing a beautiful silk slip, which was more than matched in quality by her expensive nightgown. This beautiful and very aged woman winked at me with a sparkle in her eye and said, "I may be wrinkled on the outside, but on the inside, I feel pretty."

I learned what courage and steadfast love are all about when I was privileged to be the hospice volunteer for Bob, who eventually died of Lou Gehrig's disease. He and his wife Jill made his dying as much a part of their marriage as their parenting of three beautiful daughters. During the course of Bob's illness, he had his up times and down times, but Jill and Bob never acted as if he were not still completely part of life.

Indeed, before Bob died and after his illness had completely incapacitated him, he mastered the use of a voice program to work his computer. Despite being unable to move more than a finger, he surfed the Internet collecting art and investing in stocks, and, not incidentally, he earned a nice nest egg for his family in the process.

I was deeply honored to give Bob's eulogy. During the nearly two years we were together—despite prognosis, not everyone in hospice dies within 6 months— Bob had long ceased to be simply a patient but had become a very good friend.

In my view, there can be no more important work than "being there" for people who are going through that stage of life we call dying. If you are interested in becoming a hospice volunteer, contact your local hospice organization. It is listed in the phone book.

The key person in hospice care is not the doctor, but the nurse. She visits the patient at home a few times a week—sometimes more and sometimes less, depending on the needs of the patient. When the patient has a new problem, a phone call is made to the nurse, not to the doctor. It usually takes a lot less time to reach a hospice nurse than it does to reach a doctor. She is a specialist in the nursing care of terminally ill people, and a problem that is new for the patient is usually a well-known problem to her. Many hospice nurses have "standing orders" from the doctor concerning how to manage expected problems. When unexpected problems arise, she can contact him promptly for new management orders. Since illness does not keep office hours, neither do hospice nurses. In the event of urgent need, a nurse is available 24 hours every day, each day of the year.

The nurse can function as the doctor's eyes, ears, and hands in the home. Most hospice patients are too ill to go to the doctor's office frequently, and few doctors make house calls at all, let alone several times a week. The hospice nurse is trained to assess the patient's symptoms, and to perform a physical examination pertinent to that assessment. If any new problems are discovered, they can be reported quickly to the doctor.

Most hospice staff members meet with their medical director once a week. This is not necessarily the attending physician of the patient, since most hospices take care of the patients of many different physicians. The meetings involve more than just the nurses and the medical director. The *whole team* caring for the patient works from several different angles to provide the best care possible. The hospice medical director is usually an indirect resource for the patient's care. Not being the patient's attending physician, the medical director lacks the authority to order new treatments for the patient. However, the director may be a specialist in palliative care, and, if so, can serve as a "back-up" physician to direct a new palliative intervention or to call in emergency prescriptions to the pharmacy if the primary care physi-

134

cian cannot be reached. Having a medical director on the hospice team also guarantees that patients who are relocating geographically shortly before death will be able to get ongoing medical supervision of their care.

From the Doctor's Journal:

In Tennessee Williams' famous play, *A Streetcar Named Desire*, Blanche DuBois is the character who "always relied upon the help of strangers." I often think that if Blanche had been a hospice patient, I would have been the stranger upon whose help she would have relied. My relationship with the patients for whom I serve as a hospice medical director is a curious mixture of distance and intimacy. Most of them don't know my name. A few of them remember me every night in their prayers.

I meet with the hospice team every week to discuss ongoing care of the patients. At first this took some getting used to—frankly, it was a useful exercise in humility—for me to recognize that hospice care is a team effort led by nursing concerns, not medical concerns. Still, when questions of progressive pain or other symptoms arise, I play a useful role.

One patient, I recall, was an elderly man living in a rural region far from Youngstown, Ohio. He had advanced lung cancer and had developed new pain radiating from his low back down his right leg. His nurse was excellent at her work—most hospice nurses I know are. She had gotten a detailed description of the patient's pain so that she could pass along that vital information to the patient's primary care doctor and to the other members of the hospice team. She described the pain as being like jabs of electricity intermittently shooting down the patient's leg, associated with a tingling sense in between the jabs. When

135

she had told the primary care doctor about the symptom, he had ordered a slight increase in the patient's opioid dose. I didn't think that was a very promising strategy. First, the dose increase was too little to make much difference. More importantly, the patient was already tired and constipated, and that strategy was likely to worsen those symptoms.

The pain description was classical for neuropathic (nerve damage) pain. Lung cancer frequently spreads to the lumbar spine, where it can entrap the nerves going to the leg. This man needed a treatment selected for its benefit in neuropathic pain— and he needed one that worked fast. I knew that he had only a few weeks to live. The usual therapy for neuropathic pain may take four to seven days to start working. That delay may not be significant in the treatment of a person with non-malignant pain for whom the course of the illness is measured in years, often decades. But in a dying man, those few days may be 25-50 percent of the rest of his life!

I recommended to the nurse that she ask the primary care doctor to prescribe dexamethasone instead of an opioid for this patient. Dexamethasone is a kind of a steroid. It rapidly reduces the swelling around "pinched nerves," and, therefore, rapidly reverses the neuropathic pain associated with that. For most patients with non-malignant disease, dexamethasone is *not* a good choice, because it has significant side effects over time. But I knew that in this case, we did not have to worry about long-term side effects—nor did we have the luxury of waiting for a slower drug to start working.

The primary care physician accepted our advice and ordered the dexamethasone. At the next team meeting, the nurse reported that the patient had become pain free within a day of starting the dexamethasone, and had even benefited from its side effect of boosting the appetite. He died comfortably a few weeks later. He never heard my name spoken. Frankly, that is

136

as it should be. His help came not from any one individual, but from the whole hospice *team* working together to maximize his quality of life.

◼

Patients do not need a referral from their doctors to be admitted to a hospice program. The patient, a family member, or friend can pick up the phone and call the hospice. The hospice team will then visit the patient at home to make an assessment. They will then contact the patient's physician to see if he is willing to be the "doctor of record." If the patient is an appropriate candidate for hospice care, but for some rare reason the doctor is unwilling to continue the patient's care in hospice, the hospice team can recommend another physician.

Unfortunately, too many doctors are reluctant to raise the issue of hospice—and too many families refuse to consider it—because they are afraid that the patient will be upset by the prognosis. Despite being well meaning, this reticence often does dying patients a disservice, for it deprives them of the wonderful care that hospice provides when this specialized care is, quite literally, just what the doctor ordered. Indeed, this resistance is one reason why only 15 percent of dying Americans have the benefit of hospice, compared to more than 60 percent in Britain. Furthermore, of those who do enter hospice, far too many enter care only days or a few weeks before they die. As a result, both the patients and their families miss out on months of hospice care, benefits, and support.

 From the Desk of WJS:

Too often, patients enter the hospice program too late to obtain maximum benefit. This happened to Frank, the father of my childhood best friend, a man whom I often thought of as my second dad. In 1997, Frank was dying of colon cancer. Unfortunately, it was difficult for his family to get his oncologist to agree to hospice care. When they raised the subject, he cut them off by saying that he wasn't in the business of predicting how long someone would live. The doctor's reluctance to deal with the reality of Frank's condition caused his patient much suffering.

I recall visiting Frank to pay my respects. He was clearly in agony, although he didn't tell me so. I knew because, as he talked, he would stop in mid sentence, gasping, as his eyes bulged. I asked if he was in pain. He reluctantly admitted that he was. I asked about his pain control. When I found out that his doctor had prescribed only codeine for metastatic cancer throughout his abdomen, I threw a fit! I'm no doctor, but I knew that was cruelly inadequate medicine for the task at hand.

Frank's family redoubled their efforts to obtain hospice care for him, and he was soon admitted to the nearest program. Once in hospice, his life changed from one that included intense pain and suffering into a relaxed, peaceful, pain-free ending. "Hospice was so wonderful," Frank's wife Jean told me. "I will never forget the depth of care shown by the doctor and the nurses, particularly Jill, who came every day to visit. They showed Frank such *tremendous* compassion. It is hard to believe that there are people in the world who are so deep down compassionate to strangers. But there are. They are sincere and wonderful about it."

Frank's last words to me, spoken quietly and with great dignity just three days before his death, reflected the quality of care he was receiving: "I am ready to die." No fear. No pain. Quiet acceptance.

Frank died peacefully with his family at his bedside, his favorite opera playing on the stereo. It is just too bad that he didn't benefit from months of hospice care rather than just a few short weeks.

■

The benefits of hospice for those patients who want to stop disease-directed (as opposed to symptom-directed) medical treatment cannot be overstated. The message of hospice is that each patient is valuable and important, and that dying is an important stage of life worth living through and growing from. If you or a loved one has a terminal diagnosis that is entering its final stage, please investigate whether hospice is right for you. *If your doctor does not raise the issue, don't hesitate to ask whether the time has come for hospice.*

Entering hospice is not the end of hope. To the contrary, it may be the key to helping you or your loved one transcend the physical and emotional difficulties associated with the end of life, so that life is truly lived for all of the time that remains. Indeed, it is almost a cliché among hospice workers to report that their patients have proclaimed their time in hospice a "blessing" that they would not have missed for anything in the world.

 ### *From The Desk of WJS:*

Lately, I have been receiving concerned telephone calls from around the country complaining that some hospices may not be living up to the high accolades the movement has received in this book. While I do not detect a systemic decline in quality, it may be true that some individual hospices are not as effective in their work as are others. For example, some hospices refuse to continue tube feeding of nursing home patients once they enter hospice, interpreting that as a form of life-sustaining treatment that is not paid for by Medicare. I disagree with this interpretation but know of no court or administrative rulings on the issue one way or the other. (Of course, if you do not wish tube feeding, no hospice will require you or your loved one to undergo the procedure.)

> This issue raises an important point: communication is essential to a proper relationship with your hospice providers. Thus, it is a very good idea to ask the hospice prior to entering the program about their policies on what is and is not considered life-sustaining treatment.

For those who would like more information on hospice, and to read an in-depth account of true hospice cases, we recommend the book *Dying Well: The Prospect for Growth at the End of Life*, (New York, Riverhead Books, 1997) written by Ira Byock, the former president of the American Academy of Hospice and Palliative Medicine. For more information on hospice, ask your doctor, your local hospice (they are in the phone book), or contact the National Hospice and Palliative Care Organization. See Appendix for contact information for the NHPCO.

CHAPTER 9

———■———

Potpourri

Everyone knows that cancer can be a very painful condition. No one doubts that surgery requires pain relief. But there are also many other painful conditions that may be afflicting our readers that are too often neglected in discussions of pain. In this chapter, we talk about these conditions—sincerely hoping that, in the process, we have not left anyone out—and look at the effect a person's gender and age may have on pain control.

Migraine

The very word "migraine" tells us something about both the nature of this disorder and its history. The name is derived from the Latin word *hemicranium*, which simply means "half a head." In most cases of migraine, that's where it hurts. It is a disease known not merely throughout history, but throughout the whole world. It is one of the few diseases that does not show a great variation in prevalence from nation to nation or culture to culture. It is as common in Timbuktu as it is in Tallahassee.

Up until puberty, boys are as likely to suffer from migraine as are girls. After puberty, females are much more likely than males to suffer from the disease. Thus, although a genetic predisposition seems to be a key factor in the disease, hormones clearly play a role for many patients.

Migraine is a paroxysmal disorder. That is, between attacks, most patients feel fine. *Migraineurs*, which is the lovely French name given to those afflicted with this most unlovely disease, suffer from symptoms at variable rates. About half of them have attacks less than twice a month; at least 10% have them at least once a week. Many women find a definite relationship between migraine attacks and menstruation. Women who have migraine attacks only with menstruation are said to suffer from "menstrual migraine."

For most patients, each attack is fairly similar. The headache usually affects only one side of the head, and often the throbbing pain of the headache is accompanied by nausea and vomiting. Most patients find that noise, light, or motion worsens the pain. During an attack, the typical *migraineur* is likely to be found lying perfectly still (and perfectly miserable) in a darkened room, her children having been banished to the farthest reaches of the house. Those who have suffered from both migraine and simple tension headaches say that comparing the two is like comparing lightning to a lightning bug.

Some migraine patients get a warning that a migraine attack is coming. The neurologic symptoms that may precede a migraine by hours (or rarely by a day or two) are called auras. The most common forms of auras are visual disturbances, such as seeing flashing lights, wriggly lines, or dark spots. Less commonly, the *migraineur* may experience a sudden mood change, repetitive yawning, or craving for special food. (Sorry, wanting chocolate all the time doesn't count.)

The duration of the pain is variable, ranging from 4 to a miserable 72 hours. Often patients feel enormous fatigue as the pain subsides. Whether that fatigue is a specific symptom of the illness or simply a normal response that might occur after any painful experience is not clear.

Because migraine is so prevalent, and a disease of such huge economic impact, it is the subject of vigorous research. That research has clearly benefited from the new machines that have been devised to make images of the brain. Researchers are now able to view the brain during auras and during migraine headaches. The marvelous new imaging devices, which make CAT scans seem old fashioned, can actually show changes in regional brain activity and blood flow in

142

a non-invasive way. These studies have shown that migraine attacks, both with and without auras, are usually preceded by an episode of focally diminished brain activity. For reasons not yet discovered, an area of the brain—often in the part of the brain essential for vision—becomes underactive, a phenomenon that slowly spreads to nearby areas of the brain. This is followed by a flow of activity from the brain down the nerve headed to the scalp, head blood vessels, and face. In a direction opposite to the usual flow of information, neurotransmitters are released from the nerve into the region of the blood vessels of the head. This causes the blood vessels to dilate and sensitizes them to transmit pain information back to the brain. Thus, the dilatation of blood vessels and their throbbing pain are not early events in the evolution of a migraine attack, and treatment directed at blood vessels alone, while useful, are unlikely to be completely satisfactory.

There are two aspects to the management of migraine: prevention of attacks and treatment of attacks. When attacks are very rare and not too disabling, treatment alone may be all that is required. On the other hand, the person suffering from frequent or disabling attacks of migraine clearly needs to take action to avoid them.

Let's deal with prevention first. Many *migraineurs* have been able to discover certain activities or exposures that increase their risk of an attack. Red wine triggers a migraine for some people. Inadequate rest is an even more common precipitant. Obviously, simple attention to avoidable triggers is the first step in preventing migraine attacks.

When these simple precautionary measures do not prevent the attack of pain, drug therapy may be indicated. Here, there is a wide range of drugs to consider. Probably the first one worth discussing with your doctor is riboflavin 400 mg. daily, also known as vitamin B2. This is probably the only time in this book we will recommend considering a vitamin for the treatment of a painful condition. The reason for our recommendation is that its benefit has been shown by a clinical trial comparing a placebo to the vitamin. (A placebo is an agent with no known or suspected therapeutic benefit.) In fact, this was a so-called double-blind study. In such an investigation, neither the patient receiving the medicine nor the clinician assessing his response knows whether he has received the placebo or the study drug, in this case riboflavin. It takes a few months of daily treatment for riboflavin to emerge as superior to a placebo, so a patient should not give up on riboflavin after a few days or weeks. This vitamin seems to diminish the severity, more than the frequency, of migraine. For many patients, that is enough.

Another agent to discuss with your doctor is one that is fairly well tolerated, but likely to be less effective than prescription drug therapy. That is a high dose magnesium supplement. Unfortunately, for many people, this is not a good option, since it often causes diarrhea.

Beta-blockers are a class of drugs with a wide variety of applications in medicine. They are commonly used to treat high blood pressure and heart disease, and may even be used to steady the shaky hands and tremulous voice that some people experience when speaking publicly. They are also potentially useful in preventing migraine attacks. Potential side effects (not everyone will get these side effects) include diminished exercise tolerance, weight gain, and diminished libido. The anti-epileptic agent sodium valproate has also been shown to be a useful preventive agent in management of migraine. It has a similar range of potential side effects. There are many other agents that may be useful in preventing migraine attacks. Fortunately, even when one of these drugs is not effective or tolerable for a patient, another one of them will be.

Drugs used to prevent migraine are seldom useful to treat an acute attack. At this point, it is worth quoting the sage advice in a textbook of pain medicine: "All the acute treatments of migraine are more effective if combined with a short resting period or a nap."

Many migraine attacks can be effectively treated with high doses of aspirin, acetaminophen, or non-steroidal anti-inflammatory drugs (see Chapter 2). However, because migraine attacks are usually accompanied by nausea and vomiting, many patients must take the medicine by rectal suppository and/or take it with a prescription anti-nausea medicine, which may also need to be taken by rectal suppository. Not a very elegant treatment, we admit, but the patient in the throes of a migraine attack cares very little for elegance.

When such simple measures are insufficient, the *migraineur* may benefit from one of the new drugs that have come to the market in the last few years. We refer to the class of agents called triptans that are specifically useful to treat acute migraine. For the agonized migraine sufferer, these may be true wonder drugs. A majority of patients get at least some benefit from them; many patients get quick, complete relief. Unfortunately, they are not without potential side effects. They can cause constriction of blood vessels, so they must be used with caution, if at all, by patients with coronary artery disease, or with narrowing of other blood vessels.

 ### From the Doctor's Journal:

The triptans are quite expensive drugs. But how much is pain relief worth? I learned from a desperate *migraineur* that expense can be a relative concept. When I cautioned him that the drug I was prescribing cost "an arm and a leg," he half-jokingly replied, "I don't care. It's worth it, doc. At least I'll be able to take it twice." Patients whose prescription drug expense are covered by an HMO should keep in mind that the HMO has a contractual obligation to treat them with safe, effective, FDA-approved agents for their health problems. The triptans are all of that. If the HMO doctor does not raise the subject of using these agents to manage intractable migraine, the patient should not be bashful about doing so. Sometimes doctors need a little reminder.

Public surveys have revealed that most migraine patients have never consulted a doctor about their problem. Since there is now so much that can be done to improve the lot of people afflicted with this most common of pain problems, that is truly a pity. If you are one of these people, we recommend that you see your doctor—and take a copy of this book with you.

Fibromyalgia

In fibromyalgia, we see a disease that is too often mistreated and misunderstood. Why? For one thing, the disease is hard to pin down. There is no virus or bacteria that can be detected under the microscope. No objective medical test exists that clearly proves the presence of the condition. Moreover, the victims of this chronic disorder are mostly women—whose medical complaints are sometimes not taken as seriously as are those of men. Suffering is often the consequence.

Fibromyalgia is a disease that is usually treated by rheumatologists, doctors who specialize in arthritis and related diseases. Because the disease is not fully understood, in order to foster better research, rheumatologists have come up with a complex definition of fibromyalgia so that every research report will really be describing the same syndrome. The rheumatologists' research definition describes a patient having a *specific* large number of tender points, affecting a *specific* minimal percentage of *specific* spots on *specific* muscles. It is all very *specific* (we won't bore you with the Latin names of each muscle) and very unbiological. While this definition may be useful for its purpose of establishing uniformity for research purposes, it is far less useful in the recognition and treatment of patients outside of the research setting. A more useful understanding of fibromyalgia is derived from the description the patients themselves give: *"I hurt all over."*

Although fibromyalgia patients may say they hurt everywhere, closer questioning reveals that, in fact, pain is predominantly in the muscles and their connections to the bone (ligaments and tendons).

146

Imagine how you would feel the day after you climbed the staircase inside the Washington monument, chopped down a cherry tree, stacked a cord of wood, and then, for good measure, did 100 situps and pushups. You would literally ache all over, having pain in muscles you did not even know you had. That is how the fibromyalgia patient feels every day. Curiously, many fibromyalgia patients report their daily experience with the same metaphor: "I feel like I've been beaten with a two by four."

While most fibromyalgia patients are young to middle-aged women, men also suffer from this condition. These patients go to their doctors complaining of hurting all over and of the fatigue that often accompanies chronic pain. Many of them also suffer from related invisible but distressing symptoms, such as irritable bowel syndrome or pelvic discomfort.

And this is where a patient/doctor disconnect often comes into play. Here's a patient, complaining of pain that cannot be objectively verified by x-rays or lab tests, who visibly flinches when slight pressure is applied to any muscle surface. All too often, the doctor dismisses the patient's complaints as being "all in the head," attributing them to "stress," "neurosis," "hypochondria," or all of the above.

Recently, however, researchers have discovered a biochemical abnormality in fibromyalgia patients. This may well prove to be the first wave of some major breakthroughs in this disease. The researchers have discovered that fibromyalgia patients have an elevated amount of "substance P" in their spinal fluid. Yes, that's "P" as in "pain." Substance P is an important chemical in the pain pathway. Some researchers hypothesize that the essence of fibromyalgia is "systemic hyperalgesia." Hyperalgesia, you may recall from Chapter 2, is an increased painful response from a stimulus that is usually only mildly painful. (If you're thinking, "A push on a muscle is usually only mildly painful, but, if someone had systemic hyperalgesia, then any little push or contraction of a muscle would hurt a lot," you're beginning to think like a research scientist.) The theory is that the "amplification" of the pain pathway is somehow misset in fibromyalgia, and that explains the widespread nature of the disease.

Substance P level in the spinal fluid is not a test that your doctor can order from his local medical laboratory. Substance P is a chemical whose measurement requires the sophistication of a research laboratory. We are not recommending that a spinal tap be done on patients with symptoms of fibromyalgia, and that a specimen of spinal fluid be sent halfway across the country for measurement of substance P. But just knowing about this biochemical abnormality has been a reassurance to many fibromyalgia patients who may have begun to wonder themselves if their terrible symptoms might simply be due to stress.

The management of fibromyalgia, like that of other pain problems, must be individualized. Many patients seem to benefit from a strict schedule of adequate rest, accompanied by mild exercise. Others benefit from tricyclic antidepressants used in doses too low for the treatment of depression, but adequate for many pain problems. Many fibromyalgia experts also advocate the use of opioids in some patients. If one approach does not bring relief, keep trying. All of these approaches have proven useful for various patients. What is surely *not* useful is the treatment that many fibromyalgia patients actually receive: condescension and humiliation.

Arthritis

Arthritis is one of the most common causes of chronic pain. The word "arthritis" simply means inflammation of the joint. There are many different diseases that can cause inflammation of the joints. Thus, there are several kinds of arthritis. Some arthritites (yes, that's the plural of "arthritis") are associated with symptoms outside of the joints, such as sores in the mouth or fluid around the lungs. Others affect only the joints. Occasionally, a person will have a single episode of arthritis in a single joint, and then spend the rest of his life free of joint pain. Other people are afflicted in multiple joints when they are children, and then go on to have progressive deforming joint disease for the rest of their lives.

Make Sure It's Arthritis

As with so much else in medicine, the first step to the management of this disease is a proper diagnosis. Since joint pain is such a common symptom, most primary care physicians have experience in diagnosing and managing uncomplicated cases. Unusual or severe cases are usually referred to a specialist in arthritis and related diseases, that is, to a rheumatologist.

A proper diagnosis is essential, because many of the arthritites are treated differently; some, in fact, are curable. Moreover, such discomfort can also be a symptom of a wide variety of diseases other than arthritis, including acute leukemia, gonorrhea, hemachromatosis (a disease of excessive iron storage), rubella, and drug allergy.

The diagnostic evaluation begins with the patient telling the doctor how and when it hurts. Often the patient's history gives the doctor enough information to make at least a presumptive diagnosis. This emphasizes the point we make elsewhere in this book, that smart pain patients organize their thoughts *before* going to the doctor. In the case of joint pain, the doctor will want to know which joints hurt, whether the joint pain developed suddenly or gradually, whether the patient notices stiffness in the morning. The doctor will want to know if there have been any other symptoms, such as change in vision, cough, fever, bloody nose, rash, blood in the urine, weight loss, or pain on urination. The patient should be prepared to tell the doctor what activity, if any, makes the pain better or worse.

Next, the doctor will want to examine the joints. A good doctor will also check other parts of the body, to make sure that the joint disease is not simply one manifestation of a systemic illness. Blood tests and x-rays may complement the diagnostic workup. In some cases, a definite diagnosis can only be made by the doctor's sticking a small needle into a swollen joint to remove some fluid for examination in the laboratory.

Osteoarthritis

Osteoarthritis can be thought of as "wear and tear" of the joints, such as knuckles, wrist, knee, and hip. (There is some recent evidence that this mechanical picture is quite incomplete, but the details of that evidence are beyond the scope of this book.) The cartilage that usually lines the bones in the joints is worn away in osteoarthritis. Often the patient complains of the joint being noisy as a result. As you might expect, patients who are significantly overweight are more likely to develop osteoarthritis in their knees, because those joints have been exposed to excessive load over many years. Finally, the elderly are at greater risk of osteoarthritis than are young people, due to the cumulative trauma their joints have endured.

From the Doctor's Journal:

A colleague told me the story of his examining a ninety-year-old woman whose complaint was pain in the left knee. It had developed slowly, and was unassociated with any other symptoms. On examination, he noticed her joint was noisy when he moved it, and he could feel the crepitus (crackling sound and sensation) in the joint as he moved the leg through its range of motion. The knee was slightly deformed; a layman would call it "knobby." The diagnosis was not difficult: osteoarthritis. He explained to his patient that her knee pain was due to the wear and tear of the years, that it was common in the elderly, and that there were a number of medicines that could diminish her pain. After their discussion, he gave her a prescription. She thanked him and began to hobble out of the exam room. But just short of the door, she stopped and turned to him with a puzzled look. "Doctor," she said, "the other knee is just as old...and it doesn't hurt."

Because inflammation does not play a big part in the damage of osteoarthritis, NSAIDs may not be the best choice for treatment of that disease. Acetaminophen is probably a better agent, although here too, liver function may need to be monitored, depending on the dose the patient takes regularly.

Osteoarthritis can often be relieved in ways beyond taking medicines. Many patients benefit from mild exercise programs. (Your doctor can refer you to such programs.) Obese patients with osteoarthritis of the knee do better if they are able to lose weight. When joint damage is severe, surgery to replace the hip or knee can dramatically relieve pain and improve function.

Rheumatoid Arthritis

Rheumatoid arthritis is quite a different disease from osteoarthritis, and it is often more serious. In rheumatoid arthritis, the immune system is clearly a culprit. The body acts as if joints and the tissues surrounding them were foreign invaders, so it carries on a prolonged campaign to reject the intruders. Sometimes this battle spills over, so to speak, into other areas. The immune system can cause "collateral damage" to the lungs, kidneys, blood vessels, marrow, and other organs.

Because of this fundamental abnormality, rheumatoid arthritis is sometimes treated with drugs that suppress the immune system. In years past, rheumatologists would reserve "disease modifying treatment" until the disease was fairly advanced, because the treatment carried more risk of side effects than symptom-only treatment. More recently, the philosophy has changed (because of data from clinical trials), and disease-modifying treatments are introduced early to prevent the ravages of the disease.

Fortunately, many cases of rheumatoid arthritis are relatively mild, and do not warrant such aggressive treatment. For mild rheumatoid arthritis, the non-steroidal anti-inflammatory drugs (NSAIDs) are the mainstay of treatment. Since the disease is chronic, the patient may require years of NSAID treatment. In such cases, kidney and liver function should be monitored regularly by the physician, since the drugs carry some risk of damage to those organs. In some cases, the risk of side effects, including stomach ulcers, is high enough that the doctor will prescribe the more expensive COX-2 antagonists instead of the older and cheaper NSAIDs. Frankly, not every rheumatoid arthritis patient needs the more expensive medicine. Just as frankly, a lot who would fare better with it are not receiving it.

More severe rheumatoid arthritis warrants more intensive therapy. Methotrexate, a drug that (in much higher doses) may be used to treat cancer, is clearly useful in this setting. Curiously, so are some drugs used to treat malaria. The recent introduction of monoclonal antibodies, veritable guided missiles against disease, has given rheumatologists another powerful weapon to reduce the ravages of rheumatoid arthritis.

In all forms of arthritis, specific treatment of the disease usually improves the pain associated with the disease. If that does not occur, or if pain relief is inadequate, opioid therapy may be useful. At least in osteoarthritis, opioid tolerance has not proven to be a limiting factor in treatment of pain with opioids. After a few months of mild dose escalation, most patients' dose requirements do not change, but they continue to get pain relief.

Multiple Sclerosis and AIDS

Multiple sclerosis (MS) and acquired immunodeficiency syndrome (AIDS) are diseases of quite distinct origin and pathology. But we discuss them together because they can cause similar pain problems.

MS is a progressive disease of the central nervous system. In MS, there is cumulative damage to the brain and spinal cord, charac-

152

terized by scar-like plaques in these organs. The affected areas then fail to perform normally, leading to various levels of disability. If the MS patient develops a plaque in the part of the brain or spinal cord involved with pain signaling or processing, the result can be a bothersome neuropathic pain (see Chapter 5). Sadly, there are still doctors who do not recognize that MS can be a painful illness, and want to write off the symptoms to imagination or malingering. The same drugs that are useful in neuropathic pain from other causes may be useful here. These are the tricyclic antidepressants and anti-epileptic drugs. If these fail, opioids may prove useful.

Some patients with advanced MS become paralyzed. This may result from a disconnect between the part of the brain that controls limb motion and the spinal cord. If the spinal cord is still connected to the limb, however, the patient may experience violent spasms of the limb. These may be triggered by harmful, or even harmless, stimuli to the limb. The sustained, almost violent contraction of the muscle that is the root of these spasms can be quite painful—think of a very vigorous sustained isometric exercise that's repeated too many times. In cases like this, the first step to controlling the pain is to treat the spasms. This can be accomplished with medicine that inhibits muscle contractions. One such drug is tizanidine (the trade name is Zanaflex®). It may be marvelously effective in this setting, and seldom has serious side effects.

 __From the Desk of WJS:__

      I have a close friend who has had progressive MS for many years. He isn't easily discouraged, and hasn't permitted his serious disability to keep him from his work or other life activities. Recently, however, he began to falter. When I asked why he was having a more difficult time, he told me that all of a sudden he had developed terrible pain and muscle spasms that his physician had been unable to treat. I referred him to my wonderful co-author, Dr. Chevlen, who suggested that he speak with his doctor about controlling spasms as the best way to control the pain, and then offered some ideas for that doctor to consider. My friend consulted with his doctor, who, to the doctor's credit, immediately looked into Dr. Chevlen's suggestion to see if he thought it right for this patient. Then, he wrote the proper prescription, and the spasms were quickly controlled. Today, my friend still has MS. But he is no longer in significant pain.

As almost everyone knows, AIDS is caused by a virus that attacks the immune system. If left untreated, this disease exposes the body to repeated infections that almost always leads to debility and death. (AIDS is the name given the condition when it is in its later stages.) The name of this dread virus is human immunodeficiency virus, or HIV. HIV is spread when one person's blood system is exposed to an infected person's bodily fluids, most commonly through sexual contact, sharing needles, or being transfused with tainted blood. Fortunately, the drug therapy for HIV infection has advanced remarkably, at least in developed countries, during the last ten years. HIV infection is now, for many, a chronic illness, rather than an almost certain short-term death sentence.

HIV patients are susceptible to a wide range of infections that do not usually attack other individuals. These can lead to painful complications, both due to tissue damage and neurological damage. Moreover, less known among the general public is the fact that the virus can attack the central nervous system as well as the immune system, leading to dysfunctions of the brain that are similar to those of MS.

154

Doctors treating AIDS—and persons with AIDS—must be aware of the painful complications that can occur with this illness. They must be treated just as any other painful complication of a chronic illness. For example, some HIV patients suffer from shingles. The doctor's obligation in such cases is to treat the pain just as it would be treated for any other shingles patient. People with painful conditions caused by AIDS should review Chapters 5 and 6 on chronic and acute pain, depending on the malady causing their pain.

AIDS patients who are former or current drug addicts may be more difficult to treat than those who have no history of drug abuse. Although heroin is far too short acting a drug to be a useful pain reliever, repeated exposure to it can lead to tolerance to other opioids. Thus, the drug addict may need higher doses of opioids to achieve the same pain relief that a non-addict can achieve with lower doses. Add that fact to the patient's past history, and you have a recipe for suspicion. The prescribing physician may believe that complaints of pain are really requests for assistance in getting high. A past history of drug abuse is not an absolute contraindication to opioid therapy, but it is a call for caution. If the primary doctor treating a person for AIDS is unable or unwilling to manage the patient's pain, that patient should be referred to a specialist who will treat it properly.

Sickle Cell Disease and Its Pain

This book has been written because of the pervasive problem of inadequately controlled pain in America. Racism is another problem that many, including the authors of this book, feel remains all too common in the United States. When both these problems come together, the result is often seen in the management (or mismanagement) of the pain related to sickle cell disease.

Although sickle cell disease can certainly occur in patients who have non-African ancestry, the vast majority of American sickle cell patients are black. It is a congenital disease—if you do not have it when you're born, you'll never get it. About one out of ten African-Americans is a carrier for sickle cell disease. (They are said to have "sickle trait.") Under most circumstances, carriers are free of symptoms, and may go their whole lives not even knowing they have the sickle trait. However, their children may be affected. Children of two people with sickle trait have a one in four chance of being completely free of the disease, a two in four chance of having sickle trait, and a one in four chance of having sickle cell disease.

Sickle cell disease is fundamentally a disease of the blood, more particularly of red blood cells. But because blood perfuses the whole body, sickle cell disease can have manifestations throughout the body. The normal red cell is shaped like a donut with the hole partly filled in. (Doctors refer to this shape as a biconcave disk.) The normal red cell is flexible. It has to be. As it courses from the heart to reach every part of the body, it is traveling through ever-smaller blood vessels. The final destination of red blood cells is the capillaries. These are the tiny blood vessels that are the end of the outward journey from the heart, and the beginning of the inward journey back to the heart through the veins. The capillaries are so narrow, that the red cells have to change shape a little bit to get through them. This may be compared to a partially filled water balloon being squeezed through a hole somewhat smaller than its diameter.

In sickle cell disease, the hemoglobin molecules within the red blood cell are abnormal. These molecules may be compared to children's Lego™ building blocks. A bag full of unconnected blocks can be molded into a variety of shapes. But if the blocks are stacked and connected, the bag holding them is limited in its flexibility. In sickle cell disease, the molecules of hemoglobin tend to form stacks, limiting the suppleness of the red cells. In some cases, the red blood cell gets stuck permanently in the rigid shape of a farmer's sickle, hence the name of the disease. These abnormal cells are called sickled red cells, or simply sickle cells for short.

156

If sickle cells get stuck going through capillaries, then the tissue being nourished by that capillary cannot get adequate oxygen. For unknown reasons, this blockage of flow through capillaries does not happen constantly. A sickle cell patient may go days or years between episodes. But when it occurs, it causes damage or death of the tissue involved. This can be severe, even life threatening.

As you might expect, the most likely place for sickle cells to get stuck and obstruct blood flow is where the blood vessels take sharp turns—usually where the blood vessels extend to the very ends of the bones and then make a sharp u-turn. It is no surprise, therefore, that a common complaint of sickle cell patients is sudden onset of pain in the joints.

In this book we have talked a fair bit about acute pain and chronic pain. Sickle cell pain is slightly different; it is *recurrent* pain. The sickle cell patient—they are called "sicklers" by themselves as well as by doctors—gets repeated episodes of severe pain that last for a few days to a few weeks. Each episode is referred to as a "sickle cell pain crisis." Sometimes it is difficult to know whether the patient is suffering from repeated crises, or has evolved to have a chronic pain problem from repeated injuries of the bones.

Sad to report, it is all too common that the sickler arrives at the emergency room in a pain crisis, only to meet an exaggerated form of the neglect and suspicion that many other pain patients endure. From past experience, the sickler knows what drug and what dose will relieve the pain, so he asks for it by name. The emergency room (ER) staff is confronted by a patient who is not known at all, or is known only as someone who appears repeatedly in the ER, always asking for the same "narcotics." Like other pain problems, the sickle cell crisis is often unaccompanied by any change in x-rays or blood tests. The ER doctor may suspect that the patient is faking, or exaggerating the pain. The facts that the patient and the doctor are often of different races and socioeconomic status can reinforce the gulf of distrust between them.

157

What can be done to improve this sad story of neglect, suspicion, and pain? *The best short-term solution we can recommend is for sickle cell patients to establish an ongoing relationship with a single doctor who understands how to treat pain in general, and sickle cell pain in particular.* Then, when a pain crisis occurs, the patient should call that doctor rather than or before going to the emergency room. Even if that doctor cannot go to the emergency room to the meet the patient, he or she can make a phone call to the ER doctor to establish that this patient is "legit" and to list the medications that work best for this patient.

Pain and Gender

Our earlier discussion of fibromyalgia serves as an introduction to the greater question of gender and pain. Is pain a different experience for men than it is for women? Do men and women have different "pain thresholds"? Why is it that some painful conditions are more common in women than in men?

The last question is the easiest to answer: we simply do not know. Clearly, there are many painful conditions that are more common in women than in men. In addition to fibromyalgia, migraine headaches and irritable bowel syndrome come to mind. But there are some painful diseases that occur more commonly in men, too. Cluster headache is the name of a disease with many similarities to migraine, but it occurs in men far more often than it does in women.

There are some possible explanations for why certain painful diseases strike one gender more than the other. It may be that the presence of sex hormones alters the expression of diseases. For example, in the case of migraine, we know that some women suffer from the terrible headaches only at specific times of their menstrual cycles. Obviously, their genetic makeup has not changed, and their environment is most unlikely to change on this regular basis. Hormonal fluctuations are likely culprits for this variation in disease expression. There also may be other, non-hormonal, variations between men and women that depend on differences between a woman's two x chromosomes and the man's x and y chromosomes.

But let's get back to the difficult question: Is pain a different experience for men than it is for women? Recall that pain is a subjective phenomenon. Our own experiences, and an irrefutable wealth of clinical and laboratory data, tell us that pain usually, *but far from always*, varies with the intensity of the stimulus. How can we compare the severity of pain in two individuals when we really cannot precisely compare the severity of the disease causing the pain? That is, if you wanted to compare the pain of male versus female rheumatoid arthritis patients, how could you do it? There is no precise way of measuring the severity of the disease itself, so you might be comparing the pain due to some people's severe rheumatoid arthritis with that of other people's mild cases.

Really, the only way one can compare the pain threshold or pain tolerance between individuals, or between men and women, is to do it by exposing them to a uniform noxious stimulus in a laboratory. Of course, this requirement limits the amount of stimulus that may be applied. This is science, after all, not torture. Also, it limits the type of pain that can be measured to acute pain rather than chronic pain. Since the most troubling pain problems clinicians deal with are chronic, this is certainly a serious limitation.

Another huge distinction between experimental pain and real-life pain is that experimental pain is controllable by the subject. The experimental subject knows that the noxious stimulus will stop anytime the subject requests that it be stopped. The context of pain—the situation in which it occurs and the meaning it has for the patient—has an enormous impact on the experience of pain. There is simply no way that experimental pain can truly duplicate the uncertainty, fear, and anxiety that accompany and modify the experience of pain in the real world.

Even in the situation of experimental pain in the laboratory, there are fine points of pain measurement and gender that may affect the results. For example, the gender of the researcher measuring pain tolerance may have as much influence on the results as the gender of the research subjects. To give an exaggerated example, if a pretty young female researcher is measuring pain tolerance in male college students, she may find that these fellows report less pain to her (whom they want to impress with their rugged machismo) than they would report to a grandfatherly-type researcher. Similarly, if a researcher tells the subject to report when the "stimulus" becomes intolerable, he will observe a different result from what he would have found had he asked the subject to report when "the pain" becomes intolerable.

In any event, while the differences between male and female pain experience may be important areas of research and interest for the physiologist, do they really matter that much for individual patients? If the *average* man who drops a bowling ball on his foot reports a pain score different from the *average* woman who does so, there will still be many men and women whose pain is quite different from the average. What matters most of all is that the pain be treated according to the individual's needs, and that it be relieved quickly, safely, and with respect.

Age and Pain

Like gender, age has a subtle but definite impact on pain and its management. Experiments in the laboratory show that the elderly have a higher pain threshold than the young, but a lower pain tolerance. If this statement seems self-contradictory, it is because of the precise meaning of the terms.

Pain threshold refers to the intensity at which a stimulus just begins to feel painful. A very low intensity electrical stimulus applied to the skin, for example, will not be perceived as painful by most people. But as the intensity of the stimulus is increased, almost everyone will eventually recognize the stimulus as painful. The intensity at which the change from a buzzing sensation to a mildly painful sensation occurs is the pain threshold.

160

Pain tolerance describes the other end of the pain scale. As the intensity of the stimulus increases, most people report increased pain. When the pain increases to the point that the experimental subject asks that the study be stopped, that is referred to as level of pain tolerance.

There is some decline in neurological function that occurs with age. Just as the vision and hearing are not as sharp as they were decades earlier, so the nerves dedicated to perceiving pain are not quite as limber as they were in youth. It takes a greater stimulus to activate the pain system. But once the pain is perceived, the elderly tolerate an escalation in its intensity less than do the young. The reasons for this are not clear.

One consequence of the higher pain threshold in the elderly is that they are likely to experience more tissue damage before its pain leads them to medical care. For example, stomach ulcers in the elderly are usually larger at diagnosis than they are in young people, and they are more likely to perforate the stomach before they are detected. According to experimental studies, older folks simply do not feel the pain of the disease until more damage has been done.

Pain therapy must also recognize differences between the elderly and the young. Unfortunately, chronic illnesses accumulate with age. An elderly person is more likely than a young one to have other serious health problems in addition to pain, and more likely to be taking a multitude of medications. The potential for drug interactions with other drugs increases sharply in this setting. Another fact is that many pain-relieving drugs are removed from the blood stream by the kidneys. As we age, our kidney function declines. Therefore, a dose that is just right for a young person may be excessive in an older person, since the medicine will stay in the bloodstream at higher levels and for longer time in the older person. Another distinction that comes with age is less tolerance of the sedating side effect of opioid medication. A useful rule of dosing for elderly patients is "start low and go slow."

Pain management in demented patients, such as those with Alzheimer's disease, is particularly challenging. Early in the illness, the patient can describe his pain reliably. But as the disease progresses, and the patient loses the ability to communicate, it becomes difficult to know whether the individual is in pain, and, if so, how intense it is. In this situation, the family and medical team must make their assessments of the patient's pain based on physical clues such as moaning, grimacing, restlessness, or pulse rate. It is not an ideal way to recognize and treat pain, but it is the best one available, and far better than leaving the pain untreated.

Alternative Approaches to Treating Pain

Throughout this book we have described "conventional" medical treatments for the relief of pain. Usually, although not always, these treatments involve medications such as non-steroidal anti-inflammatory drugs, opioids, or other drugs. For a variety of reasons, some people prefer to avoid these approaches and, instead, try non-medical approaches.

Hypnosis

There is no question that hypnosis can play an important and useful role in some cases of both chronic and acute pain. But there is an enormous question as to what that role is. As the noted pain researcher Patrick Wall has emphasized in his recent book, *Pain: The Science of Suffering* (Columbia University Press, 2000), the pain perception system is not simply one nerve connected to another like links in a chain. All along the pain pathway there is input from the brain. The brain is able, in many cases, to amplify or reduce the intensity of the pain signal racing up the spinal cord to the brain. More importantly, these descending influences from the brain, as well as pain reducing activity within the brain itself, can lessen the pain experience, not just the intensity of neurological activity in the spinal cord. Hypnosis is one of the techniques of taking conscious control over pain perception.

162

Many patients have learned to achieve the benefits of hypnosis with no formal instruction. They may call it "tuning out" or "focusing elsewhere," but the result is the same. Perception (of pain) is absolutely essential for the full pain experience. If patients can "turn their attention" elsewhere, at the expense of perceiving the painful stimulus, the pain experience can be reduced. The reader may complain, "But isn't that simply ignoring pain, and not really getting rid of it?" Keeping in mind the absolutely subjective nature of pain, we would reply, "What's the difference?" By that, we do not mean, "What difference does it make to you which technique you use to reduce pain?" We mean something deeper. We mean there is no meaningful distinction between pain (completely) ignored and its absence. In either case, power has been exercised over pain.

Not everyone can use hypnosis, and not every person's pain is lessened by it. In our experience, mild to moderate pain is more readily relieved by hypnosis than is severe pain, but we recognize that "clinical experience" is not the same thing as scientific proof. Like any other therapy, the patient considering hypnosis should weigh the potential risks and benefits. Its risks are quite small, but not zero. They are the risk of wasted financial resources, the risk that it simply won't help, and the risk of wasted time and prolonged suffering before finding a more effective therapy. Possible benefits may include pain reduction with no drug side effects, and avoidance of the expense of drugs or surgeries. Without better clinical research, this may be the best advice we can give.

Acupuncture

It is ancient. It is mysterious. It is Eastern. But is it useful? Questions swirl around the subject of acupuncture. We'll try to make some sense of it.

Acupuncture is a method of pain relief based on the insertion of needles into specifically defined areas of the body. Whether or not the original theory underlying it—a theory based on such mystical

163

concepts as yin and yang, and meridian lines—is accurate is of secondary importance. Theories are useful for proposing testable hypotheses, and for organizing a wide array of information into a logical pattern. Whether a theory is right or not does not change the validity of the data.

Perhaps an example from the history of medicine will clarify that concept. Decades ago, an Australian researcher noticed that rodents exposed to a significant quantity of lithium in their drinking water behaved in a much calmer manner than did rodents drinking regular water. He theorized that the lithium had a specific calming effect, and proposed that it would be useful in treating humans afflicted with mania, a psychiatric disease characterized by excessive agitation and flight of ideas. His hunch was wonderfully correct, and, to this day, lithium remains an important treatment of mania and bipolar disorder (a disease in which episodes of mania alternate with crippling spells of depression, commonly known as manic-depression). As for his original theory concerning the rodents, it was flat-out wrong. It turned out that the rodents were not calm; they were intoxicated. While lithium can normalize the thinking and behavior of manic humans, the dose used on the rodents was simply bludgeoning their brain function. In fact, they were being poisoned by that dose of lithium, and their apparent calmness was due to the fact that they were just plain sick.

Let's get back to acupuncture. Keep in mind that there is a big difference between a bogus theory and a worthless treatment. Therefore, when we state that we do not believe the original theory underlying acupuncture, that does not mean that acupuncture is necessarily worthless. Similarly, when we propose a more modern theory explaining why acupuncture should work, that does not mean that the treatment is necessarily useful. In science, data, not theory, rules.

The Western theory underlying acupuncture is consistent with numerous other experiments. We know that there are different types of pain nerve fibers in the skin and other tissue. One type is the C-fiber. It seems to be responsible for transmitting information interpreted as dull, achy pain. The A-delta fiber, on the other hand, transmits information interpreted as being sharp, prickly pain. The next time you pinch your finger in a drawer, you'll be able to feel the difference in the fibers' function. The sharp jab of pain you feel when your finger is pinched is brought to your brain courtesy of the A-delta fiber. The achy throbby pain that arrives a second later, and does not go away for a while, reflects the activity of the slower C-fibers.

When we shake, rub, or blow on the injured finger we are applying a technique that underlies the theory of acupuncture. In essence, we're trying to stimulate the A-delta fibers, since we would rather feel their messages than those of the C-fibers.

Yes, often it seems it is either/or. Either we feel the sharp, prickly pain effect of the A-delta fibers or we feel the dull, achy pain effect of the C-fibers. The modern theory behind acupuncture is that needling stimulates the A-delta fibers, and that their stimulation leads to a blockade of signals from the C-fibers.

But this theory does not tell us whether acupuncture really works. To answer that question, we must return to the difficulties associated with scientific pain studies. We need to compare acupuncture to *something*, but to what? If we simply compare the pain scores of chronic pain patients treated with acupuncture to those who are on a waiting list to receive it, we run into several confounding factors. First, the acupuncture group received *something*, while the waiting list group received *nothing,* or (worse, from the point of view of the research) a variety of self-selected pain therapies whose dose, duration, and complications are unknown to the researcher. That is an open door for a huge placebo effect favoring the acupuncture group. Second, the acupuncture patients received an ongoing, and frankly uncomfortable, therapy for a significant period of time. They are emotionally invested in the results; they *want* it to work. This too will affect the outcome of the study.

From the Doctor's Journal:

In the context of clinical practice, this patient invest-ment in the outcome may actually be useful. I have noticed a similar phenomenon in my work. As my practice has grown busier, there is a longer waiting time, sometimes a few months, before chronic pain patients can be seen. It is perhaps no coincidence that the success rate with treating chronic pain has been rising as my practice grows busier. While I would like to think that it's because my skills are improving steadily, I also recognize that patients waiting a long time to see a doctor—I don't mean a long time in the waiting room, but a long time between the call for the appointment and the appointment it-self—build up a perhaps unjustified expectation, based on the theory that anyone this busy must be darn good at what he does. It may be that part of the therapy's benefit is the non-specific effect of heightened patient expectations. Mind you, neither my patients nor I are complaining about this.

So, to what should acupuncture be compared? Some studies have compared "real" acupuncture to "sham" acupuncture. In the latter, needles are inserted into areas of the body that are thought to be inactive in the benefit of acupuncture. Fortunately for the study subjects, but unfortunately for the research, needling of these sham sites might not be as inert as once thought. It may be that, despite the lovely diagrams of acupuncture sites illustrated with exotic Chinese characters, the benefit of acupuncture, if any, does not depend that much on where the needle is stuck.

Another problem with the studies on acupuncture is that the sheer number of patients studied is too small. Again, a comparison will clarify the concept. Let's say that a friend of yours claims that by "mind power" he can control the flip of a quarter—with your quarter, and you doing the flipping—to be heads or tails. You tell him that you'll give him the quarter if he can prove it. He says he'll make three heads in a row occur, and sure enough, that's exactly what happens. But that really proves nothing. Mere chance, rather than mind control, is the more likely cause of the quarter landing heads-up. On the other hand, if your friend could make the quarter come up heads a *hundred* times in a row, it would be difficult to dismiss his claim.

In published acupuncture research on chronic pain, most of the studies have too few patients or insufficient control groups for us to draw any definite conclusions. They are like the quarter flipped to heads three times in a row. Keep in mind, too, that researchers are more likely to submit small studies showing a benefit of a therapy than they are to submit similar studies showing no benefit. This is called publication bias.

Interestingly, it turns out that the poorer the design of the acupuncture study, the more likely it is to conclude that acupuncture is useful in the treatment of chronic pain. Now that does not prove that acupuncture is worthless. Absence of evidence is not evidence of absence. But the best we can conclude about acupuncture for chronic pain is that there is limited evidence that it is better than no treatment at all, and inconclusive evidence that it is more effective than placebo, sham acupuncture, or standard care. All that being said, however, if acupuncture helps relieve your pain, then what difference does it make to you how or why it works? Let the scientists work it out while you enjoy a more comfortable life.

Alternative Therapies

How about other "alternative therapies" for pain, such as homeopathy, herbs, vitamins, or "therapeutic touch"? Here the list is long, and the data are short. The question of alternative therapies is inevitably intertwined with the question of the placebo response. This requires some explanation.

A placebo, you will recall, is an agent with no known or suspected therapeutic benefit. It is often used as the control arm in a randomized study. For example, if aspirin were just discovered this year, and we wanted to know if it were useful for relieving the pain of, say, toothache, we would take a hundred patients with toothache, and give half of them aspirin and half of them a similarly-shaped pill containing lactose, or corn starch, or a similar agent assumed to be of no benefit.

The interesting point is that many patients experience a definite benefit from the placebo. This may be how some alternative therapies seem to help some patients. They think it will reduce pain, so it does. Still, there may be more going on. Strangely, some studies have found differences among placebos, with patients reporting better pain relief from red placebos than from yellow ones! In any event, with regard to alternative treatments, about all we can conclude is whether a treatment is better than placebo or equal to placebo. Of course, a therapy may even prove worse than a placebo if it actually causes harm.

Undoubtedly, much of the claimed benefits of alternative therapies are from their placebo effect. It is conceivable that some of the therapies may actually be better than placebos, but that remains to be proven scientifically.

 __From the Doctor's Journal__:

When a patient asks me about an unproven therapy, I usually explain that it is untested, and, therefore, we simply don't know whether it works. I try to judge the safety of the proposed treatment. For some treatments, the safety is easy to judge. For example, if a patient asks me whether putting a bar of soap under the sheets will prevent night time leg cramps, I reply that I have no reason to think so, but that I can see no harm and little expense in trying. On the other hand, patients who ask about herbs such as St. John's wort must be cautioned that it contains a potentially toxic ingredient, while those contemplating going to the Philippines for "psychic surgery" must be advised that they would be throwing away a considerable amount of money for a treatment of no proven benefit.

Sometimes patients, speaking of alternative therapies, will tell me, "Well, at least it can't hurt." I ask them how they know. A treatment that has not been assessed for benefit has also not been assessed for harm. That a treatment is "natural" is no automatic protection. Even vitamins have been proven to worsen some conditions.

But aren't some "standard therapies" also of unproven benefit? Strictly speaking, yes. There are many therapies commonly used today that have not been tested by clinical trials. That is why the practice of medicine is as much art as it is science. That is why there is no substitute for an honest, experienced doctor.

It is amazing, not to say alarming, how many patients decide on a treatment based simply on the recommendation of a stranger they meet at a grocery store, or an article they read on some web site. These same people would not let an amateur fill out a tax form for them, but will entrust their health to uninformed advice. The tax code may be monstrously complex, but it is simplicity itself compared to the workings of the human body. If you would not let an amateur advise you on one, why let him determine your care of the other, especially considering the potential for harm that untested substances can cause the body?

CHAPTER 10

———■———

Pain Control & Health Insurance

For too many people, health insurance issues limit pain control treatment options. "What kind of health insurance do you have?" is the first question many patients hear when going to see a new doctor. This is obviously a crucial question. Medical treatment is expensive, and most people cannot afford the full cost of care.

Different countries have developed different approaches to paying for health care—none of them totally satisfactory. In England, for example, medicine is socialized, with taxes paid to the National Health Service footing the bill. However, socialized medicine has resulted in long waiting lines and deterioration in the quality of care, only partially remedied by a private insurance system permitted by law to pick up the slack. Canada has a national health insurance system, paid by the national government and each province, in which private sector physicians treat patients. This system—similar to Medicare in the United States, but available to the general public—has both its plusses and minuses, including cheaper medications but longer waits for treatment.

Then we have the hodge-podge system in the United States. Here, there are three forms of paying for medical services: "cash or charge?", private insurance, and government insurance. Pain control, as a legitimate medical treatment, is generally covered by both government and private insurance, and of course is accessible for uninsured patients who can afford to pay as they go. For the uninsured without the means to pay for themselves, access to quality pain control, like access to other forms of treatment, may be as illusory as the search for a pot of gold at the end of a rainbow.

170

Private Insurance

Most people pay for their health care through private insurance. This is often provided as part of an employee's compensation package. Individual insurance policies are also available at market prices, but they can be very expensive. The high cost of insurance is one of the major reasons why approximately 44 million Americans do not have health insurance coverage at any given time.

Fee-for-Service Plans

Up until the last decade, most health insurance policies were "fee-for-service" plans. As the name implies, fee-for-service means that the insurance company pays the doctor, hospital, etc. a fee for every covered medical service you receive. Under this type of policy, you or your doctor submit bills to the insurance plan, listing the procedures performed or the dates of hospitalization, and the insurance company pays for the portion it is obliged to pay under the terms of the policy.

Fee-for-service plans are divided into different sections. The first is usually hospitalization. This type generally covers the following expenses:

- A semi-private hospital room and bed; (If it is medically necessary for you to have a private room, that too will be covered, but such situations are the exception rather than the rule.)
- Routine nursing care;
- Hospital food (such as it is);
- Use of the operating room or other special facilities if medically necessary;
- Minor medical supplies;
- Lab tests, x-rays, and other medically necessary diagnostic procedures;

- Doctors' bills incurred as a result of surgery or hospitalization;

- Outpatient care if connected with the surgery or the accident that caused the hospitalization.

There are several things to look out for in your hospitalization coverage:

- How much of the total bill is covered? The best policies pay the entire tab, but not all do.

- How long does the coverage last? Some policies set a time limit for paying benefits, typically 120 days.

- Is there a waiting period before benefits kick in? Most hospitalizations aren't of sufficient duration to exhaust benefits, but some policies require the patient to pay for the first several days of hospitalization, which is not kind to the pocketbook.

- What is excluded? Like any insurance policy, what the policy appears to give on one hand, it may take away in the other. Many hospitalization policies do not cover hospitalization for convalescent care, for example.

- Perhaps most importantly, are preexisting health conditions covered? Many policies exclude from coverage, at least for a time, hospitalizations required by medical problems that were present before the start-date of the policy.

The second major coverage in a fee-for-service policy is major medical. The primary purpose of major medical benefits is to provide protection during illnesses, prolonged treatment of illnesses, or other serious medical conditions.

There are generally three distinct features about which you need to be aware in a major medical policy:

172

- What are the maximum benefits? Unlike most managed care contracts, to be discussed below, there is a dollar limit to the total that major medical coverage will pay, both yearly and over the duration of the policy. Obviously, the more money you have in the pot the better you are protected.

- What is your deductible? The key feature in a fee-for-service contract is that, before the insurance company has to pay any money for your care, you must pay a predefined amount called "the deductible." (Typically, this is $250, although to save money on premiums, many people select higher deductibles.)

- What is your co-payment? The other key feature of a fee-for-service contract is your responsibility to pay a proportion of the costs of your care after the deductible has been exceeded. (Most contracts have the insurance company picking up 80 percent of the cost of care and the patient paying 20 percent, with a maximum annual payment by the patient, generally around $5,000.)

A key issue for pain patients in fee-for-service health insurance contracts is whether the cost of medications is covered. Some provide such protection; others do not. Therefore, prior to obtaining this kind of insurance, including a PPO (see below), check whether the policy pays for prescribed drugs, and learn whether there are limitations in the policy that may reduce that benefit.

The PPO

The quality and variety of medical interventions available to save lives and relieve disease has grown enormously in the last several decades. And higher quality in medicine, as in everything else, usually carries a higher price. A new Cadillac costs more than a used Ford. The essential difference between health care and automobiles, however, is that many people are content to drive a used Ford, preferring to put their limited economic resources in another area. But when it comes to health care, no one is willing to settle for what they see as second best.

The fee-for-service type of insurance plan got caught in the squeeze between the rising cost of health care and the virtually unlimited demand for it, among other issues that combined to increase costs. Thus, the price of this type of insurance rose dramatically over the years to the point where many people can no longer afford it. As a consequence, pure fee-for-service insurance has to some extent gone the way of the horse and buggy. In order to permit fee-for-service insurance to remain viable and affordable—certainly a relative term in this context—the insurance industry developed a hybrid form of insurance known as the preferred provider organization (PPO).

A PPO tries to save money on both ends of the equation. By contracting with a limited number of physicians, hospitals, and other medical "providers," it reduces the price it pays for services. (The doctors, hospitals, and other service providers agree to accept a lower level of compensation from the insurance company. In return, the insurance company refers patients to them as authorized providers of the PPO.) And, by creating a number of barriers to limit patient demand, or at least access, for a number of services, the PPO reduces the number of medical events for which it must pay.

In many ways, a PPO works like traditional fee-for-service insurance. There are deductibles, co-payments, and coverage divided between hospitalization and major medical. But the PPO also combines a few of the characteristics of managed care (see below), the form of health insurance that is quickly becoming the primary approach to health care financing in the United States today. For example, managed care restricts the doctors whose services will be paid for to an approved panel, a constraint that does not exist in traditional fee-for-service insurance. A PPO, on the other hand, offers greater coverage for services that are provided by approved physicians and hospitals than if the medical care or testing is provided by a physician or institution that is not a member of the PPO panel.

Thus, there is a significant financial incentive for patients to use approved providers. However, unlike pure managed care, the insurance will pay for services provided by non-approved doctors, but at a substantially lower rate. For example, your co-payment if you go to a plan-approved doctor may be 20 percent, but it may be 40 percent for a non-approved physician. Similarly, if you are hospitalized, there will likely be a significant difference in the amount your insurance company will pay if your hospital is PPO-approved as opposed to a non-approved hospital. Also, like managed care, you will usually need advanced approval for some services, otherwise the treatment is on your dime or you receive substantially lower coverage—even if you use an approved provider.

Perhaps the most significant impediment you will face as a pain patient in a fee-for-service plan, including PPOs, is whether your request for pain treatment is considered usual and customary and/or medically necessary. If it isn't, the company doesn't have to pay. And guess who decides whether the treatment is necessary. (Right. It sure isn't you!)

As a way of keeping an eye on the bottom line, your insurance company is likely to have a medical review department looking over your doctor's shoulder. If this committee disagrees with your doctor's approach to your care, either in its necessity or its approach, the committee may disapprove your claim. In such cases, your doctor may have to go to bat for you, or you may have to fight your insurance company for coverage.

The HMO

In the last ten years, there has been a profound revolution in health care financing that has turned the controlling economics of medicine upside down. That revolution has a name: managed care. The primary structure of managed care is the health maintenance organization, better known by the three letters, HMO.

This brings us back to fee-for-service medicine. Up until the managed care revolution, fee-for-service governed the economics of medicine. It encouraged physicians and hospitals to provide services, and plenty of them, since the more that was done for a patient, the more money was made. Eventually, for a wide variety of causes beyond those mentioned above and beyond the scope of this book, pure fee-for-service medicine became too expensive, and "cost containment" became the watchword of the era. That led to changes in health care financing, both from government sources and private insurance. These changes are still sending shock waves throughout the medical professions. HMOs are now the most important form of health care financing in the country.

An HMO finances health care through a payment system known as capitation. That means you or your employer pays a fixed premium to the HMO, in return for which you are entitled to receive all the health care you need (or at least all the health care the HMO thinks you need, which may be quite a different thing), including preventive services, with very little further money coming out of your pocket. For example, a doctor's visit in an HMO may cost you $5 or $10, while under a PPO plan you might have to pay the entire tab if you have not already met your deductible.

What's the catch? Good question. If you join an HMO, in all but life-threatening emergency situations, you must use *only* the doctors and facilities authorized by the HMO. In other words, in return for lower premiums, no deductible, and scant co-payments, you give up some freedom of choice in health care.

This lack of freedom sometimes causes intense problems for pain patients. It may be difficult to get a referral to a pain control specialist, a matter of far less difficulty in a PPO or fee-for-service plan. Much of this has to do with the capitation system. HMOs induce your doctor to provide the bulk of your care through financial inducements. This is done through "positive" incentives, such as providing bonuses for having an "efficient" practice, and "negative" incentives, such as threatening the doctor with loss of income or participation in the HMO contract—or both. These incentives are designed to induce your doctor to either treat you personally, or refer you to only physicians who are members of your doctor's group practice. (Because of financial pressures, most doctors who have HMO contracts participate in large group practices of about 50 or so doctors of varying specialties, known as an independent physicians association, or IPA.)

This is where pain patients may be behind the proverbial 8-ball in HMOs. IPAs will always have physicians who are board certified or qualified in common specialties such as cardiology or surgery. Unfortunately, many do not have a pain specialist as a member. In such cases, you may have to fight your insurance company (and perhaps your own doctor) for an authorized referral outside your primary care physician's group or beyond the HMO's overall approved panel. There is some good news about HMOs, however, that partially compensates for these shortcomings. Unlike some fee-for-service plans or PPOs, managed care insurance generally covers the entire cost of prescribed medications over and above a modest $5 or $10 co-payment. This is wonderful—at least on paper. Unfortunately, what the HMO gives with one hand, it may partially take back with the other.

In order to control their costs, most HMOs create a list of approved medications for particular conditions. Often, these are the ones that are the least expensive and/or perfectly fine for most patients, but which do not work well, or are associated with intolerable side effects in a minority of patients. The approved medications list, called a formulary, is an effective tool in managing financial resources. If an HMO will not cover unlisted medicines—even if your doctor specifically prescribes them as the best treatments for you—then resource management ceases to be prudent stewardship and, instead, becomes a straightjacket that limits your doctor's ability to treat you effectively. In short, when this happens, cost containment becomes a polite term for degrading the quality of care.

Whether you have fee-for-service insurance, PPO, or HMO coverage, you may have difficulty obtaining payment for your pain control. Getting around these restrictions may prove troublesome, so you should pay very close attention to your insurance company's dispute resolution processes. (These will be spelled out in your policy.) You should also not hesitate to enlist your doctor's help in educating your insurance company as to why the particular course of treatment is necessary in your case. Unfortunately, this also may be problematic since some doctors are reluctant to engage in frustrating bureaucratic arm-wrestling. This is not merely because this time is uncompensated. Many times the doctor wants to avoid the irritation and insult of being kept on hold, only to have his medical judgment challenged by someone at a distant 800 number who has neither seen the patient nor, for that matter, the inside of a medical school. These are vital issues for any pain patient. Your doctor's willingness to fight the insurance bureaucracy on your behalf may be the difference between obtaining the best pain control and achieving second-rate palliation. In worst case scenarios, your only out from this "Catch-22" is to sue.

If you have a seriously painful malady or injury, having good health insurance is almost as important as having a good doctor. As we have seen in this brief discussion, each form of coverage has its plusses and minuses. You will have to decide the kind of coverage that is best for you—least expensive (generally HMOs), or the insurance with the most depth, a comprehensive fee-for-service plan. Whichever type of coverage, in these days of cost-controlling medicine, you may or may not run into an insurance problem. If you do, be ready to fight aggressively for the medically warranted pain control you deserve.

From the Desk of WJS:

Getting into a dispute with your HMO is a stressful, upsetting endeavor—and that's when you prevail. Lose and the consequences can literally be life threatening.

The key to obtaining the care to which you are entitled in such disputes is your willingness to break through the roadblocks HMOs erect in your path to simply wear you out. An excellent resource in this regard is the short but helpful book *Fight Back & Win: How to Get Your HMO and Health Insurance To Pay Up*, (Bottom Line Publishing, Greenwich, CN, 1998). The author is William M. Shernoff, an attorney who has forced many a health insurance company to their knees for failing to pay proper benefits. Included in the book are discussions of how to get your insurance to pay benefits, overcoming roadblocks, insurance traps to avoid, HMO coverage for Medicare recipients, and answers to the nine most commonly asked coverage questions.

Government Insurance

The three primary forms of government insurance are Medicare, Medicaid, and veterans hospitals and clinics. Medicare is federally financed insurance that covers senior citizens and a few other groups, such as people with disabilities or people who need dialysis for kidney failure. Medicaid is a form of health care financing co-funded by the states and the federal government. It is intended to provide a safety net for the poor. Medicaid coverage varies from state to state, but must meet a minimum standard defined by the federal government. The Veterans Administration provides health care for some, but not all, veterans. In this book, we will restrict our discussion to Medicare and Medicaid.

Medicare

For most people age 65 or older, Medicare is the only health insurance game in town. The program is similar to fee-for-service medicine, coming in two parts: hospitalization, known as "Part A," and major medical, cleverly and imaginatively called "Part B." There is no direct cost to Medicare beneficiaries for their Part A hospitalization coverage. Other than that, it works generally like a traditional fee-for-service policy. There is a substantial deductible, which slowly increases each year. After you have paid the deductible, you receive complete coverage for the first 60 days of your hospitalization. If you must remain in the hospital after 60 days, you have a co-payment responsibility for the next thirty days. (Contact your local Social Security office for the current deductible and co-payment figures.) After that, you are on your own during each benefit period, except that you are permitted 60 reserve days in a lifetime, to which you can turn if you have one of those very rare extended hospitalizations.

In order to reduce costs, Medicare pays for your care through a system known as DRG, diagnosis related group. Here's how the system works:

- When you become ill, your doctor diagnoses what is wrong. This diagnosis becomes the basis for determining whether you are entitled to benefits with hospitalization, paid only if the hospitalization is medically necessary. As we shall discuss immediately below, the diagnosis also affects the level of compensation paid by Medicare to the hospital.

- In some non-emergency cases, your doctor must submit a request to Medicare to get permission to admit you to the hospital before surgery, or other inpatient medical treatment. This requirement is waived if the delay in treatment, while waiting for approval, would harm you.

- The hospital will be paid a lump sum payment depending on your diagnosis (DRG). Let's assume you are diagnosed as

180

having a medical problem—we'll call it Disease X—which requires hospitalization. Medicare bureaucrats have already determined how long, on average, a person with Disease X remains in the hospital. Let's assume that is 5 days. In that case, Medicare will pay for five days worth of care (or at least for what they determine should be the price of five days of care), whether you spend 2 days or 12 days in the hospital.

The financial incentive created by DRGs is obvious: *the sooner you leave the hospital the better for the hospital.* Think about it. If you leave the hospital after 2 days, the hospital is paid for five days worth of care, three of which they did not actually provide. That means more financial benefit for the hospital. On the other hand, if you are hospitalized for 12 days, the hospital loses money by having had to provide you with 7 days of care, which, from the hospital's perspective, is provided to you for free. This may lead to some patients being pressured to leave the hospital before they may actually be ready to do so.

You will know if the hospital wants you to leave when you receive a written document called the Notice of Noncoverage. Receipt of the document does not mean that a pair of burly hospital orderlies will appear to remove you bodily from your room. But it does mean that the continued cost of your hospitalization will be on you after the Notice of Noncoverage becomes effective—no small or inexpensive matter.

If you believe that your discharge would be harmful to your health, you have a right to appeal the Notice of Noncoverage. Here are some of the measures you can take to protect yourself or a family member if such a problem should arise:

- Ask your doctor to assist you. Hospitals depend on their doctors on staff (those authorized to admit patients into the facility) to stay in business. Thus, doctors have some clout, *power* that can in some cases make the difference between a too-early discharge and those few extra days that can mean so much to a complete recovery. Your doctor's assistance in this regard is crucial because *it is against the law for the hospital to try to get you released before you are medically ready.* Thus, your doctor's assertion of the potential harm of discharge will be a major part of your case for continued coverage.

- Get copies of your medical records. Patients in most states are able to obtain copies of their medical records. For people living in these states (approximately 40 as of 2000), the primary issue you will face is the cost associated with obtaining your records. While a few states require that patients be allowed free access to records, most allow the hospital or doctor to charge a reasonable cost for reproducing and mailing your records. If that is a concern to you, you should ask the doctor or hospital what the cost would be before ordering your records.

If you live in one of the states without an explicit legal right to obtain copies of medical records, that doesn't necessarily mean you will be denied access. However, if your request is refused, you should contact an attorney to see whether litigation might do the trick. You might also consider contacting your local state or federal legislators for help since elected office holders often are able to open doors that private citizens cannot.

If your treatment was provided in a federal hospital or other federal health care facility, you should be able to obtain your records without significant difficulty, since the Federal Privacy Act generally gives you the right to "review" your records "and have a copy made..." Any refusal of your request must be made within ten days. In the unlikely event you have to sue to obtain your records and you prevail, you are entitled to the recovery of reasonable attorney's fees, costs, and perhaps money damages against the federal government.

- Appeal the decision if you or your doctors do not agree with the Notice of Noncoverage, and informal attempts to gain extra time have failed. You must appeal if you wish to remain in the hospital on Medicare's dime. Once the appeal is filed, you will be dealing with an administrative entity known—brace yourself for another acronym—as the Peer Review Organization (PRO). Don't procrastinate! Once you receive your Notice of Noncoverage, you will only have two days of Medicare-paid hospitalization left. Happily, you can start the appeal process by simply picking up the phone and asking the hospital operator to give you the phone number of the PRO.

If you appeal and win at the PRO, part or all of the extra hospitalization will be covered by the Medicare payment to the hospital. If you lose, any time spent after the two days will be on you. Of course, you also have the right to seek redress in the courts if you are unhappy with the PRO decision. (Some lawyers specialize in cases such as these. Just as you are better off with a cardiologist if you have heart disease, you are more likely to prevail in court if your lawyer is very familiar with the rules surrounding Medicare and Social Security.)

Medicare Part A covers some services outside of a hospital as well, and this may be relevant to the treatment of pain. If you need inpatient nursing care at a skilled nursing facility *after a hospitalization* and the condition for which you need care *is the same one that was treated at the hospital, P*art A may pay for the first 20 days of care and pay part of the costs for the next 80 days. In some circumstances, Part A may also pay limited benefits for in-home health care services, such as intermittent skilled nursing, physical therapy, medical social services, and durable medical equipment. Perhaps most importantly in the area of pain treatment, Part A covers hospice treatment, a wonderful form of care for people who are dying that is described more fully in Chapter 6.

Medicare Part B, unlike hospitalization, is not a completely tax-supported coverage. However, the premiums are so modest that Medicare major medical must surely be the best buy in town. Most people elect to have their premium deducted from their Social Security checks.

In order to obtain coverage, you must actively enroll in the program. This is not as simple as it sounds. Medicare is not an open enrollment program. To make sure you are not left out in the cold, be sure to contact the people at Social Security well before you become eligible for Medicare for an explanation of how the system works.

Part B is similar to the major medical coverage provided by fee-for-service insurance plans. If services are medically necessary, Medicare will help pay for part of the cost of care. Services such as surgery, outpatient hospital care, diagnostic tests, and other forms of treatment, such as oncology, pain control, and diagnostic physical exams, are covered. With a few exceptions, such as mammograms, Medicare does not generally pay for preventive care. There is a modest deductible.

Here is a list of covered services under Part B:

- Outpatient hospital care
- Ambulance services
- Durable medical equipment
- Administered drugs
- Outpatient therapy
- Chiropractors
- Second opinions

Note: *At present Medicare does not cover prescribed medications,* a major issue when it comes to most methods of pain control.

Benefits are paid on the basis of what is called a "reasonable charge." This much is sure: the "reasonable" charge will almost always be less than the amount the doctor actually bills. Moreover, Medicare *only pays for 80 percent of the "reasonable" charge,* regardless of the actual physician's fee. You are responsible for the balance. Thus, if your doctor charges you $500 for a procedure, and the reasonable charge allowed for the service by Medicare is $300, you are on the hook for the $200 difference plus $60 (the 20 percent co-payment of the $300 reasonable charge), for a total patient responsibility of $260—roughly half of the actual fee. Moreover, you must pay the entire $500 fee to your doctor and then apply to Medicare for reimbursement of its share of the bill.

You can reduce your financial obligation and the personal hassle of seeking reimbursement by going to a doctor who agrees to "accept the assignment." By accepting the assignment, the doctor agrees to accept payment directly from Medicare. This means you do not have to make the entire payment in advance. More importantly, in return for receiving direct payments from Medicare, the doctor agrees to accept the reasonable charge as the actual charge for the procedure. Thus, in the case above, you would only have to pay the $60 co-payment rather than $260—a substantial saving.

Why should doctors accept assignment if it means that they will have to write off so much of their usual charges? Medicare purposely created several incentives to make sure many doctors would accept assignment. First of all, accepting assignment reduces the risk that the doctor will receive nothing at all for his services. An auto dealer may be able to repossess the car that was not paid for, but what can the doctor do if the patient does not pay for an appendectomy—put the appendix back in? And, since Medicare requires that the issue of accepting the assignment be an all or none deal, the loss of money is compensated by the doctor not having to chase down people in lawsuits for unpaid fees.

Medicare publishes a list of doctors in your area who will accept the assignment. For a copy, contact your local Social Security office.

Filling in the Gaps

From this discussion it is clear that, while Medicare is very helpful (particularly since many people who qualify for Medicare would not qualify for private insurance on their own), it provides incomplete protection—both financially and in terms of coverage—for many patients. This applies doubly to pain patients who must use prescribed medications to treat their conditions. Fortunately, there are some actions you can take to fill in these gaps.

- Join an HMO: As noted above, HMOs have prescription benefits and do not require expensive deductible or co-payments. Moreover, you may elect to convert your Medicare benefits to HMO coverage. In such cases the government pays the HMO, and you rece*ive benefits from that plan.* Be aware that this means you are no longer entitled to the Medicare benefits we described earlier, but must either receive your medical care through the HMO or pay for it yourself. Unfortunately, after sweeping into the Medicare market a few years ago, many HMO companies are now pulling back from the senior citizen market. They found that the Medicare reimbursement was not high enough to cover the cost of treating the population that had elected HMO coverage. Thus, it may be difficult to find an HMO willing to accept you as a Medicare patient.

- Purchase "Medi-gap Insurance": Many private insurance companies sell policies to fill in the benefit gaps (areas where Medicare does not fully pay) and/or coverage gaps (areas in which Medicare offers no benefits). The government does not sell medi-gap policies, but it does regulate the industry. As a consequence, all medi-gap insurance companies sell

186

fairly standardized policies, which will vary in terms of benefits and price. If you are in the market for this insurance product, be sure to carefully compare the benefits offered, premium cost, and potential exclusions, *most particularly whether the medi-gap policy covers the cost of prescriptions.*

Medicaid

The other major government insurance is Medicaid, a federally aided, state operated program of health care assistance for the poor. The federal government and the respective states co-fund the program.

Each state is allowed to make its own rules concerning what is and is not covered by Medicaid, subject to some very loose federal guidelines. Because each state has different rules, you will have to contact your local state human services office to check coverage and eligibility requirements in your area.

In general, Medicaid covers the following for eligible recipients:

- Inpatient hospital or skilled nursing facility care;
- Outpatient hospital services;
- Laboratory and X-ray services;
- Doctor's services;
- Home health care;
- Some transportation to and from medical care.

These are the basics. Many states provide more. Some will pay for eyeglasses, dental care, prescription drugs, and other services.

The major catch to obtaining Medicaid is that patients must usually spend down their assets almost to the bone before being allowed into the program. There are sometimes ways around this requirement, particularly for married couples. Indeed, "elder law" attorneys specialize in helping people plan for Medicaid by arranging their assets and affairs to permit "asset preservation." People entering their senior years are advised to consult an elder law attorney for estate planning, including asset preservation and other services such as will writing, creating advanced medical directives, etc. They should not wait until they are sick to get this advice, since some asset preservation plans require years to take effect.

 From the Desk of WJS:

While this is a book about pain control, a word or two about advance medical directives is definitely in order. An advance medical directive is a legal document by which you create written instructions designed to control the course of your own future medical care in the event you are unable to make health care decisions.

There are two primary types of advance directives—the "Living Will" and the "Durable Power of Attorney for Health Care." There are also hybrid documents that combine elements of the Living Will with those of the Durable Power of Attorney for Health Care.

The wording of these documents is crucial and could make the difference between whether you receive medical treatment or have it withdrawn. Be wary of Living Wills (also called "declarations" or "directives"). They give doctors the power to decide whether treatment is to be provided to you: not necessarily a good idea in this age of cost-cutting and managed care. Also be warned that many "form" advance directives that are given out by hospitals upon admission are almost exclusively aimed at refusing care rather than discriminating between the types of treatments you would want and those you would wish to forgo.

A Durable Power of Attorney for Health Care in which you appoint someone (often referred to as an agent or health care representative) is best. The reason is that no document alone can contemplate every possible contingency. More importantly, by appointing someone you trust and who understands your values, you increase the likelihood that the decisions made about your treatment and care will be consistent with decisions you would have made had you been able.

A good, state-specific advance directive for those who wish to assure that their desires regarding the provision or refusal of medical treatment are carried out is the Protective Medical Decision Document (PMDD), provided by the International Task Force on Euthanasia and Assisted Suicide. The PMDD is a Durable Power of Attorney for Health Care that allows you to appoint a person you know and trust to make health care decisions for you in the event that you are temporarily or permanently unable to make such decisions for yourself. The PMDD contains a provision that actions not be taken to intentionally end your life. It also directs that, whatever you decide regarding curative or life-sustaining treatment, you always receive optimal pain control. For more information on the PMDD, see the Appendix.

If You Do Not Have Insurance

If you want to obtain pain control and do not have insurance, you are in a tricky, not to mention painful, spot. Still, there are a few tactics you can use to find relief.

- Pay for it yourself. Some doctors will accept monthly payments if you cannot afford to pay as you go. However, some will want substantial or full payment for all services rendered.

- Explain your financial circumstances to the doctor and ask that the charges be waived, in other words that the doctor treat you for free. While many doctors will decline this opportunity, some will appreciate the patient's frankness. Of course, be prepared for questions from the doctor, like "How can you afford to buy cigarettes but cannot afford to pay me?"

- Try to find a teaching hospital to provide your care. Doctors who will be treating you there are fairly new graduates from medical school but work under the supervision of senior physicians. Ironically, some of these interns and residents are more up to date on the newest treatment options than the doctors who have been in practice for many years.

- Many drug companies offer free medication to people who cannot afford to buy their products. Your doctor may know about some of the programs, but do not depend on this. Ask your doctor or pharmacist for the name of the drug manufacturer's representative in your area, and contact that person directly.

Paying for pain control treatment is almost as important as the treatment itself. This chapter has attempted to give you sufficient knowledge about this important issue to help you to begin maneuvering effectively through the various health care financing systems. However, just as books on medical problems cannot substitute for a doctor's assessment, so this chapter is not intended as legal advice. If you or a loved one find yourself in a situation in which payment for pain treatment is denied by your insurance, you should consult a lawyer to determine your rights.

CHAPTER 11

■

You & Your Doctor

Clearly, your doctor is the most important person in helping you exercise power over pain. The importance of this relationship cannot be overemphasized. A good physician/patient relationship increases the chances that the patient will receive optimal care. Conversely, when the patient and doctor are not in sync, the result is often less quality medical care, which may not hurt the doctor, but can definitely hurt the patient.

Ideally, patient and doctor should operate like a good dance team, whose partners move together to create poetry in motion. Another good analogy is that of a business partnership. Just as business partners have the common goal of earning money, a doctor and patient's common purpose is excellent medical care. And just as different partners may have different jobs to perform on behalf of the partnership, patients and doctors have different tasks that each must fulfill if the overriding purpose of their relationship is to be fulfilled.

That is not news. Nor will it be a shock to most readers when we state that, far too often, physicians and patients act as if they are not on the same team. When this happens, the patient's care may limp weakly forward when it should stride confidently ahead. If the common goal of the physician/patient relationship is the relief of pain, it is the patient who suffers most when the partnership is not working as it should.

That being so, you and your doctor should do everything possible to ensure that your partnership will be productive and cooperative. Toward that end, this chapter will deal with the duties your doctor owes you, as well as the responsibilities you have toward your

191

doctor (a topic that is often neglected in books of this type). These are actually two sides of the same coin. Remember, the overriding goal of the partnership is to maximize the quality of your health care. When your doctor does right by you and you do right by your doctor, the beneficiary is you.

Your Doctor's Duties

Your doctor is your fiduciary, a legal term that describes a special duty that one person owes another, based on a family, legal, or business relationship. One of these special relationships is that of doctor and patient. Your relationship with your doctor is different than the one you may have with your local dry cleaner or plumber. Those business relationships are known as "arms length" transactions, in which the service provider is not under a special duty of loyalty or care. That is not true of the physician's relationship with you. Under the law and the canons of medical ethics, your doctor, as your fiduciary, owes you the *highest* duty of loyalty, excellence, and responsibility. This duty is so high that the doctor must, in many circumstances, put you first, even above his or her own financial interests. The duty applies whether or not your medical problem is pain, cancer, a physical examination, or plastic surgery.

This is not a legal treatise, and so we will not attempt to teach you the law of fiduciaries. However, the following responsibilities are consistent with your doctor's solemn responsibilities toward you, the patient.

Proper Qualifications

Every licensed physician has the legal right to treat any patient for *any* health condition. That does not mean, however, that every doctor *should* do so. After all, obstetricians may be excellent at delivering babies but may know little about plastic surgery or new medical breakthroughs in treating back pain. In other words, for each medical condition, not all doctors have equal skills.

This is especially true when it comes to treating pain. As we stated previously, too many doctors in this country are woefully undertrained in pain control. And, even given good training, some doctors have better skills than others. Some have a greater interest in the subject of pain management than others, and a greater commitment to achieving pain control for the patient. And while it is true that most doctors can treat ordinary and transitory pain (pain that is not severe or long-lasting), many simply do not have the ability to treat chronic or severe pain, which is an entirely different biological entity.

Of course, just because a doctor is not adept at pain control does not mean that that individual is not a fine physician. After all, no doctor can know everything, which is why medicine has been divided into various specialties and subspecialties. Still, *if your doctor does not have the ability to handle your pain problem adequately, he or she has the fiduciary obligation to tell you so.* In such cases, you should be referred to a doctor who is an expert in the treatment of pain, just as you would be referred to a proper specialist if your medical problem were heart disease or cancer.

Confidentiality

Health care is a very private matter. Not only is it extremely personal, but also what others know about our health can, and sometimes does, hurt us. Doctors and society have recognized this fact all the way back to the ancient Greeks and the famous physician Hippocrates. Indeed, part of the Hippocratic Oath obliges physicians who take it to keep their patients' confidences.

Confidentiality is clearly an important matter when it comes to the treatment of pain. First and foremost, it is nobody's business but yours (and those to whom you choose to share your medical condition) that you are suffering from a painful condition. Second, since there is often no objective test to prove or disprove the existence of pain, some pain patients suffer under the false assumption of others

193

that they are hypochondriacs or that their physical problem is actually psychological or emotional. Then, there is the fact that some pain must be treated with opioids, which have another name in a different context—narcotics. As discussed in Chapter 4, it is unfortunate but true that some ignorant people do not make a distinction between the proper medical use of these drugs and the abuse of these substances.

(There are a few exceptions to the right to confidentiality in medicine. If you sue your doctor for malpractice, your medical history may become an issue in the case. If you have a "reportable condition," such as tuberculosis or a sexually transmitted disease, your doctor is obliged to notify the local health department. Your right to confidentiality to the rest of the world still applies, unless you have signed a release permitting the doctor to provide your medical information to insurance companies and other third parties. As with any important documents, *you should carefully read release of information documents before signing them.* Your insurance company may also obtain this information when your physician seeks payment for services rendered.)

You Decide

Up until the last twenty years or so, when a patient was under a doctor's care, the doctor, not the patient, decided the kind and duration of medical treatment. Thankfully, those days are long gone. Today, it is the *patient* who has the ultimate right to accept or reject medical testing or care. This is known as the right to "informed consent."

Having the right to decide means little if you do not have the information necessary to make a proper choice. Under the doctrine of informed consent, it is your doctor's solemn obligation to tell you the pros and cons of each test and each plan of treatment. This includes the purposes for the procedure or prescription, the anticipated benefits and risks, as well as the alternatives, if any. The doctor also should offer recommendations as to how to proceed, and the bases for those recommendations. However, in the end, you have the right to decide how to proceed.

This obviously holds true in the treatment of pain. In any medical act, there is an up side and a potential down side. For example, if you suffer from chronic pain and your doctor recommends an opioid, the hoped for positive result is obviously the effective treatment of your pain. But there will also be other factors to consider: the cost of the medication, constipation and the need to combat it with laxatives; the risks of drowsiness and physical dependence; and the potential, even if highly unlikely, of other or severe unanticipated reactions. Upon being told the entire story—both positive and negative—you then have the right to decide whether to proceed with the treatment of your pain. Your doctor's job is to use his or her training and expertise to present you with the various options, and then to proceed with the course of care that you have accepted.

The Right to Know What Is Going On

Once you have given your informed consent to proceed with treatment, you have the right to know what is happening with your care, step-by-step. For example, if you have decided that your back pain is best treated with the surgical insertion of a spinal pump, you are not only entitled to know the plusses and minuses of the pump, and the benefits, risks, and alternatives of surgery, but you also have the right to know *what is going to happen to your body* each step of the way. You have the right to be told about the anesthesia that will be used during surgery, what you can expect to feel during the procedure, and what it will be like for you after surgery. The doctor may tell you, "You will feel exhausted and sleepy. If you feel sick to your stomach, don't be alarmed, but be sure to tell the nurse," etc.

Protection of Your Dignity

There are few times in life when we feel more vulnerable than when we are being examined or treated by a doctor. This being so, part of your doctor's obligation to you, the patient, is to minimize this potential discomfort by preserving your dignity and sense of proper decorum. For example, you have the right to draping if your examination or treatment requires you to disrobe. Women being treated by a male doctor have the right to the presence of a female nurse or attendant in the examining room. You have the right to have your privacy preserved and protected by having examining doors closed. You have the right to expect that your doctor will retain a clinical demeanor that does not cause you embarrassment or undue alarm. And you also have the right to be addressed as Mr., Mrs. or Ms., if you prefer that, rather than by your first name.

The Right Not to Be Abandoned

Once a doctor has undertaken your care, you cannot be abandoned. This right may mean many things. For example, if you are being treated for a heart attack and your insurance company refuses to pay benefits, the doctor can't just leave you on your own with a life-endangering condition, but must continue necessary care even if he or she is not paid. However, prior to the initiation of care, a doctor is under no legal obligation to accept you as a patient. What's more, the doctor can discontinue the physician/patient relationship for any reason not prohibited by law, or even for no reason at all, so long as it does not constitute abandonment during a time of needed treatment. Many pain specialists ask their patients to sign "contracts," acknowledging that the doctor will discontinue the relationship if the patient is found to be abusing or diverting (illegally selling or distributing) controlled substances.

In summary, the doctor may not simply terminate your care abruptly. If you are informed by the doctor that he or she no longer wants to be your physician, you must be given a reasonable period of time, usually about a month, to find another doctor. You cannot simply be thrown to the wolves without access to needed care.

Non-abandonment also means that the patient must have access to care whenever it is really needed. Your doctor must be available in an emergency. It also means that, if your doctor is away, there is an "on call" physician available to accept urgent calls and provide care in situations that cannot wait. In short, if you need care, your doctor or an "on call" substitute must be accessible. This also applies to any doctor who is treating your pain.

Respectful Treatment

Part of being an empowered patient is to refuse to put up with behavior by doctors or their staff that is insensitive, discourteous, or disrespectful. Respect, of course, means different things to different people. But here are some constants. You have the right to:

- Prompt return of telephone calls;
- Reasonable waiting times before an office visit;
- Neat and clean waiting and examining rooms;
- No interruptions with the doctor, absent an urgent matter;
- Your doctor's full attention to your concerns;
- Respectful treatment by physician and staff.

The behavior you receive from your physician and staff in non-medical areas may be an indicator of the quality of medical care you receive. If you are not treated respectfully, you may wish to find another doctor.

Keeping Up to Date

One truth about medicine is that it is constantly changing. That is why a good doctor's education is never completed. Part of his or her job is to take continuing medical education classes and to read the medical literature (articles in medical journals) that update readers on new medical developments. If you ever come to believe that your doctor does not take this need for ongoing education seriously, the time may have come to find a different doctor.

Referral to a Specialist

There was once a time in medicine when the general practitioner knew almost everything there was to know about your treatment. Those days are long gone. Medical knowledge is now so broad and deep that no single human being can keep up with every development.

That is where medical specialization comes in. Many medical conditions can be treated effectively by your primary care physician, usually an internist or a family practitioner (both of whom are medical specialists in their own right). However, if your medical problem is beyond the expertise of these physicians, they will generally refer you to what is known as a "sub-specialist," that is, a doctor who has in-depth training and experience in a narrow area of medicine. Thus, if you have a significant heart problem, your internist will refer you to a cardiologist, who is an internist with a subspecialty in diseases of the heart. Likewise, if you have metastatic cancer, your doctor will refer you to an oncologist, who is an internist with special training in the medical treatment of cancer. Some diseases even require the super-refined skills of a sub-sub-specialist. For example, there are doctors who specialize just in diseases of the retina or in the management of patients with transplanted organs.

Most specialties are determined through a process known as board certification. For each area of practice, medical boards exist that determine the training and experience required to become "board certified." Once a doctor has completed this training, he or she is "board eligible," that is, the physician is now a proper candidate for certification. To actually become board certified, a doctor must successfully pass a rigorous written (and sometimes oral) examination. To learn whether a doctor is truly a specialist in your area of concern, the proper question to ask is usually not, "Are you a specialist?" or "Are you board eligible?" but rather, "Are you board certified?"

Pain control and its modern advances are a relatively new area in medicine, and there is not yet a single board that is recognized as *the* accrediting body for this specialty. There are at least three boards with overlapping areas of interest in the field. It is expected that in the next few years, there will be a clarification of the relative role of each. The American Board of Pain Medicine certifies physicians who demonstrate specialized training and knowledge in the field. The American Board of Pain Management (not Pain Medicine) will also extend their certification to non-physicians. The American Board of Anesthesia offers a subspecialty certification in pain management for anesthetists who have demonstrated the requisite level of competence. Realistically, there is some political jockeying for turf among these three boards. But, all other things being equal, a doctor who is certified by any one of them is likely to have better knowledge of treating pain than a doctor who is not. So, if your doctor—whether your primary care physician, oncologist, or other specialist—is not successful in treating your pain, you should be referred to a medical specialist in the treatment of pain, hopefully one who is properly certified and trained in this new and exciting field of medicine.

Access to a Second Opinion

Doctors are people too, meaning that sometimes they make mistakes, or they may simply be inadequate to a task. The problem, of course, is that medical mistakes and inadequate physician knowledge can hurt you. That is why a patient must feel free to get a second opinion if he or she is not comfortable with the doctor's diagnosis or recommended courses of treatment, or if the diagnosis is sufficiently serious that extra assurance of accuracy is needed.

Anytime you believe that your doctor is not serving your best interests, you should consider obtaining a second opinion. A second opinion can do much to clear the air. It can demonstrate that you and your doctor are already on the right path. It can help add extra brainpower to a problem that your doctor is finding difficult. Look at it this way: either the second opinion will concur with the first, giving you more confidence in it, or it will disagree, giving you a valued new outlook. (Of course, when the two opinions differ, there is no guarantee that the second one is the better.)

If you are like many patients, you may be worried about offending your doctor by asking for an extra pair of eyes and ears to review your case. Do not be. If your doctor becomes angry or hurt by your request, then you may be with a doctor who is more concerned with his or her own ego than with your health. In such cases, you are probably better off finding another doctor. If your doctor can walk on water, do not get a second opinion. Otherwise, it is worth considering.

Optimal Care

The right to optimal care means that your doctor is duty-bound to do the best possible job attending to your health care needs regardless of your age, race, sexual orientation, gender, personality, or any other factor. Another aspect of receiving optimal care is related to the issue of qualifications, discussed earlier. Under the professional duty to render optimal care, your doctor is obligated to let you know if he or she is not properly trained or experienced to deal with your pain problem. After all, there is no shame in recognizing one's limitations and referring you to a doctor who can give you the level of care you need.

What are the danger signs that you may not be receiving the best care that is available to treat your pain? Here is a partial list of danger signs:

- Your doctor does not give high priority to the treatment of your pain;
- You are in pain after receiving pain treatment and your doctor tells you there is nothing more to be done;
- Your pain is not adequately treated within a reasonable time;
- You keep having unanticipated setbacks in your pain control or you experience side effects about which you were not forewarned;

200

- Your doctor tells you that *you* are the problem, that the problem is all in your head, or that your complaints are exaggerated;

- Your doctor cannot answer your questions about pain management, such as what to do about side effects or what alternative pain control treatments can be tried if initial attempts prove unsuccessful;

- Your doctor resents you wanting to be intimately involved in your own health care decisions;

- Your doctor resists a second opinion;

- Your doctor is unavailable to answer your questions or grapple with concerns;

- Your doctor is in poor health and unable to focus appropriately on your medical needs;

- Your "sixth sense" is telling you things are not right.

Part of exercising power over pain is not settling for second-rate medical treatment. If you find that your doctor is not providing you with the level of care you deserve, especially after you have discussed your concerns, it may be time to find a better doctor.

Your Responsibilities to Your Doctor

A productive and beneficial relationship with your doctor is a two-way street. Just as the doctor has professional duties toward you, you in turn, have obligations toward your doctor. The idea behind these patient responsibilities, of course, is not to benefit your doctor so much as to maximize your doctor's opportunity to help you.

Communicate, Communicate, Communicate!

Like any partnership, the patient/doctor relationship requires open communication if it is to thrive. We have already addressed your

doctor's obligation to fully inform you about your own health condition and any recommendations for future care. But you also
have substantial communication responsibilities in this regard.
After all, your doctor is not a mind reader and can only work with
the information you provide. To put it another way, what your
doctor does not know can hurt *you*.

Communication is especially important when it comes to pain.
There are several potentially harmful consequences if you fail to
be completely candid with your doctor about whether and how
you are hurting. First, as discussed earlier, pain is one of the body's
primary ways of alerting you that something is wrong. Failure to
describe your pain fully and accurately can lead to your doctor's
failure to properly diagnose what's wrong. Second, failing to tell
your doctor fully and completely about your pain can cause your
doctor to give or withhold treatment that would otherwise have
been provided (or avoided) had the full story been known. Third,
your doctor is not going to care more about your pain than you do.
If you keep quiet about your pain, do not expect your doctor to
lose sleep at night worrying about whether your pain keeps you
awake.

Good communication is a skill. It takes forethought and care.
We are not saying that you have to act as if you have a medical
degree, of course. You do not have to use fancy Latin terms or big
words to get your point across. You merely need to be descriptive,
candid, and thorough when informing your doctor about your pain.

Assume you are being treated for cancer. You develop pain
in your stomach that gets worse after you eat, but which slowly
goes away over several hours. At its worst, the pain is not so bad
that you are doubled over from it. However, it is significant enough
that you are always aware of it while it lasts. If your doctor is to
deal with the pain and its cause, you have to say exactly what is
going on. Here is a *wrong* approach:

202

Doctor: So, John, how are you feeling?

Patient: Not bad, Doc. A little indigestion, but it always goes away.

Doctor: Indigestion? What do you mean?

Patient: It's no big deal. Probably heartburn or gas. I've been taking Tums® and that seems to help.

Doctor: You're sure you're okay?

Patient: Yeah. If it gets worse, I'll call you.

This scenario is not at all unusual. Too often, patients underreport their pain. Perhaps they fear that, by admitting their pain, it means a previously diagnosed illness has worsened, or maybe they merely want to be "good" patients by not bothering their doctors with matters they do not believe are serious, based on a misguided self-diagnosis. Some don't want to know what they don't want to know.

But "hiding" the existence or extent of pain is a prescription for suffering. It is also dangerous because it may deflect your doctor from following up, ordering tests, or referring you to a different doctor. And while it is true that most doctors would (hopefully) not be as willing as the doctor in the above example to let the matter rest, in today's increasingly time-pressured medical environment, some doctors would. As a consequence, not only might available pain relief not be made available to the patient, but quite possibly, a serious physical condition would go undiagnosed.

Now, compare the above hypothetical with this better approach to communicating about pain:

Doctor: So, John, how are you feeling?

Patient: I have pain in my stomach after every meal.

Doctor: What kind of pain?

Patient: Well, it's not like I was kicked in the stomach. It doesn't double me over. It feels more like I have a bruise. But it comes on every time I eat and always in the same place, right here (pointing to his breastbone). On a scale of one-to-ten, ten being unbearable pain, I give it a three.

Doctor: So, it's more of a dull pain than a sharp one?

Patient: Right. I've been keeping track. It usually lasts for about three hours after I eat and then goes away by itself. This has been going on for about two weeks. I tried Tums® and that seemed to help reduce the intensity but it doesn't make the pain go away.

Note how much more the doctor knows from the patient's second discussion than from his first. The doctor now knows exactly *where* it hurts, the *quality* of the pain (such as sharp, dull, burning, etc.), its *intensity,* its *duration,* and that an over-the-counter medication does not eliminate it. Perhaps most importantly, the patient does not push the doctor away from investigating the pain, as he did in the first conversation.

What Your Doctor May Ask You About Your Pain

- ✓ How did the pain begin?
- ✓ Where does it hurt? How long has it hurt?
- ✓ Does the pain radiate anywhere else?
- ✓ How intense is the pain?
- ✓ Does the intensity of the pain vary? What makes it better or worse?
- ✓ What is the quality of the pain? (For example, burning, prickly, jabbing, throbbing, etc.)
- ✓ What therapies have been tried? What benefit did they have? What side effects?

✓ Have you seen other doctors for this problem? What did those doctors do or say?

✓ Are you involved in any litigation concerning this pain?

✓ Are you allergic to any medicines? What reaction did you have that makes you think you are allergic?

✓ Do you have any other ongoing health problems? Have you had any serious health problems in the past?

✓ What medicines are you currently taking?

✓ Have you ever had any addictions to alcohol or other drugs?

✓ What impact does the pain have on your ability to perform activities of daily living, or your ability to earn a living?

✓ What impact has the pain had on your personal relationships?

✓ What impact has the pain had on your mood?

✓ Are you depressed? Have you had thoughts of hurting yourself?

✓ Is the cost of prescribed medicine a barrier in treating you?

Be Prepared

If communication is the backbone of an effective physician/patient relationship, then you, as a patient, should be prepared to do your part to make the interaction with your doctor fruitful and productive. Now, some may think that is obvious. It isn't. Many patients go to their doctors and, for a variety of reasons, are unprepared to communicate effectively about their condition because they do not prepare properly for their medical consultation.

Lack of patient preparation can be a serious matter. After all, your doctor's ability to assist you is, in large part, dependent upon your providing all of the information your doctor needs to do a thorough and competent job. If you are unable to provide the data, or if you actively withhold information, you are impeding your doctor's ability to treat you properly.

What does it mean to be a prepared patient? A prepared patient is one who compiles information and brings it to the doctor's office ready for use. The following is a list of things your doctor will probably want or need:

- **Written "talking points."** When politicians communicate on television, they rely on "talking points," a list of arguments that they want to make to ensure that the message they seek to communicate is the actual message that is put out. Similarly, when you go to the doctor, it is a very good idea to *write down ahead of time* the issues you wish the doctor to address and bring the list with you to the appointment. In that way, nothing will be missed, and your treatment will not be delayed.

- **Your medical records.** Obviously, if the doctor who is treating your pain is your primary care physician, that won't be an issue. But if you have been referred to a specialist or are consulting one on your own, you need to make sure that your family doctor forwards relevant copies of your medical records so that there are no gaps in information about your condition and course of treatment.

- **A list of all your medicines.** It is essential that you disclose all of the medications you are taking to your doctor. Many of today's medicines are powerful chemical agents that have a profound impact on your body. That, of course, is the point. But if you are taking other drugs—even over the counter medications, vitamins or herbal supplements —they may alter the chemistry and/or efficacy of the drugs, and may even cause a toxic effect. Do not simply try to memorize the names of your medicines. Write down the names, the dose, and the schedule of your taking the medicine. Even better, grab all your medicine bottles, throw them in a paper bag, and bring them with you for the doctor to review.

206

- **A list of all your doctors, past and present**. This can be important since a key part of your doctor's job in diagnosing and treating you consists of taking a good "patient history." This consists not only of a list of your ailments, but also when those conditions occurred and what was done about them. The simple truth is that, as time passes, many of us forget this information, and your current doctor may need a source to call to fill in any gaps in the essential information. It is also a good idea to have a list of any hospitals to which you were admitted in the event your doctor needs that information.

- **Insurance records**. American medicine being, well, American medicine, the first question you will be asked when you walk through your doctor's office door is, "Do you have health insurance?" To prevent delays in your care, be sure to bring your health insurance card, Medicare card, or other proof of insurance to every office consultation.

- **Translator**. If you have difficulty with English, be sure to bring a translator with you to prevent miscommunication.

 From the Doctor's Journal:

The usefulness of the patient's bringing the medicine bottles along on a visit was brought home to me in a powerful way. I was treating a young woman for the pain of metastatic melanoma. The aggressive skin cancer had spread to her liver, bones, and throughout her skin. When I had first met her, she had been in a lot of pain, but, with steady increases of her morphine dose, she had become comfortable and more able to interact with her husband and young children. I saw her in the office, and I was pleased with how well she was doing. I wrote a new prescription of her sustained-release morphine tablets, and asked her to see me again in a few weeks.

But just a few days later, her husband called to tell me that she was having a virtual crisis of pain, associated with chills, abdominal cramps, nausea, and diarrhea. I knew that this was not something I could handle by telephone, so I asked him to bring her into the hospital for evaluation and treatment.

As I examined the patient, her husband remarked that she seemed to have gotten worse right after she started the new blue pills I had prescribed. "What blue pills?" I asked. I distinctly remembered that I had **not** made any change in her medication. "These," he said, handing me the bottle.

I looked at the label. It indeed read MS-Contin® 200 mg., just as I had prescribed. But wait a second, I thought! The 200 mg tablet isn't blue; it's gray. I opened the bottle, and there I found the blue pills the husband had referred to. The pharmacist had labeled the bottle correctly, but had put 15 mg. tablets in it, rather than the prescribed 200 mg. tablets. No wonder she was in pain! Her dosage of morphine had suddenly been reduced over 12-fold. Not only was the 15 mg. dose completely inadequate to control her pain, but she was in acute opioid withdrawal as well. Had the patient and her husband not brought the bottle of pills into the hospital with them, it would have taken far longer to discover the cause of my patient's problem.

Ask Questions

Your doctor is highly educated and trained. That's the good news, of course. Proper education and training are key ingredients to providing medical excellence. But there is a downside to all of the information contained within your doctor's cranium. He or she may speak an obscure and arcane language used primarily by doctors and research scientists, known as "Medicaleze." Medicaleze is not a language that most patients easily understand. In Medicaleze, for example, most words have multiple syllables. And while, technically, Medicaleze is English (with much Latin thrown in), most of the words are not those studied by people who are not health professionals. For example, if you are told that your pain has "an idiopathic etiology," what your doctor is actually saying is, "I don't know why you hurt."

This brings us back to the importance of communication. Part of your job as a patient is to understand what your doctor tells you. Hopefully your doctor will explain matters in a way you can understand. But if that does not happen, it means *you* should ask for a better explanation in words you recognize. This advice does not solely apply to pain control, of course, but to any medical issue. When it comes to understanding your own health care, the old cliché holds true: there are no stupid questions.

Follow Your Doctor's Advice

Once a course of treatment for your pain has been agreed upon, *follow it.* If you have been prescribed one pill every six hours, do not take two pills every twelve hours; do not take three pills a day; do not take the pills only if you hurt. Take one pill every six hours.

You should also take your prescription for as long as you are directed. This is particularly important when recovering from surgery or some other cause of acute pain. In those cases, stopping your pain-controlling medicine too early may lead to pain and the need to increase your medication to get it back under control.

If the doses that the doctor has prescribed are inadequate to control the pain, do not simply take more. That may be dangerous for you, depending on the drug. Also, doing so will make the doctor worry that you are abusing the medicine he has prescribed, and that will make him reluctant to prescribe more. The best thing to do is call the doctor's office to report the failure of the drug, and ask if it is OK to take more. That will reassure the doctor that you are still working together as a team, rather than striking out on your own.

Do Not Delay Reporting Your Pain

Your doctor is willing to work hard for you, five days a week, and, when necessary, on weekends and holidays. Still, doctors have lives, too, and they want to spend time with their families and in other non-professional activities, just as everybody else does. That is why doctors hate "Friday Afternoon Specials," in which patients who get sick on Tuesday wait until Friday afternoon before reporting their problem to their doctor.

This is equally true when it comes to pain control. If you are being treated for pain and you are in pain, do not delay informing your doctor. This is important information that your pain control specialist needs to adequately provide the palliative care you desire. What's more, by the time you find that you can no longer "grin and bear it," you may find that your doctor is unable to squeeze you in at the last minute—meaning that you may spend extra days in pain. Also, if you need tests to determine the future course of action, labs may not be able to return test results (assuming it is not a life endangering emergency) until after the weekend.

Of course, we are not saying that if you need your doctor on a Friday, Saturday, or Sunday, you should not call to protect your doctor's home life. If your doctor is not available, there will be a doctor "on call" to take care of your needs. Keep in mind, however, that the "on call" doctor is there just for emergencies, and probably does not know your case well—or, perhaps, not it at all. This doctor's role is simply to care for you until your doctor is again available, not to make adjustments in the long-term plan that you and your doctor have devised. What we are saying is that, if you are a pain patient and experience a loss of palliation, call sooner rather than later. That is best for your health and helps your doctor provide you with the best possible care.

Tell Your Doctor How You Feel

Part of your responsibility as a patient is to tell your doctor how you feel, both physically and about the way you are being treated as a patient.

On a physical level, your pain doctor needs to know if the treatment is working. Your doctor does not want a "yes patient" any more than you want a doctor who only tells you what you want to hear. As we discussed earlier, if you are still hurting, speak up. If you are experiencing side effects, let your doctor know. If you feel something is not quite right but cannot quite put your finger on the problem, maybe your doctor can. Of course, if the treatment is working, your doctor needs to know that too. That is the joy of medicine: helping people regain their health or, if that is not possible, helping them feel better or become free of severe pain.

You should also make a point of telling your doctor if you are satisfied with the way you are treated as a patient. If your doctor's staff has impressed you with their courtesy or professionalism, tell the doctor and give them a boost with their boss. If not, spill the beans. After all, your doctor's business is serving people, and if there is a glitch in the system, he or she has a right to know. Besides, telling your doctor is a lot easier on your nerves than changing doctors because you cannot stomach the staff.

This advice goes double for matters directly concerning your doctor/patient relationship. Too many of us are in awe of doctors and tend to treat them with kid gloves rather than speak the truth (politely, of course) and let the chips fall where they may. Such timidity is not doing you or your doctor a favor. Remember, your doctor is not a mind reader. Problems cannot be solved unless they are brought up.

So, if you are unhappy with your doctor for any reason, schedule a meeting to clear the air. We'll bet that your doctor will be anxious to resolve the difficulty. And, if not, it is better to learn sooner rather than later that your doctor does not care enough about your business. In any event, you'll sleep better at night once the problem is out in the open.

A related issue to speaking your mind is showing appreciation. We have become so used to medical "miracles" and scientific break-throughs that we tend to forget how hard our doctors worked to learn the healing arts, and how hard they must continue to work to keep current on the latest techniques. So, when your treatment is success-ful, let your doctor know how grateful you are, and how much better you feel. A thank you card, a box of candy, or maybe a plant to spruce up the waiting room in recognition of a job especially well done is likely to be a courtesy that spreads geometrically throughout your doctor's practice. After all, there's nothing like unexpected recogni-tion to add gusto to one's work. If you are cured of an illness and no longer need to see the doctor, or if you no longer see him because he has corrected your problem and returned you to your primary care doctor for ongoing care, send him a Christmas card to let him know you're still doing well. It brightens the whole office to get such greet-ings and reminders of success.

Be Considerate of Your Doctor's Time

While it is certainly true that too many patients are forced to cool their heels in a doctor's waiting room, we must remember that con-sideration of time is a two-way street. Thus, just as you have the right to expect your doctor to be prompt in seeing you at the appointed time, you should be as considerate of your doctor's time schedule. This is also a matter of politeness to your fellow patients. One or two tardy patients early in the day can throw an entire day's schedule out of whack.

212

When you think about it, this responsibility is not very tough; it is simple courtesy. Here are some suggestions:

- Be on time for your appointment, and call if you are going to be late. Your doctor may be able to fit in another patient early, and keep the day's schedule flowing smoothly.

- Restrict your appointment to the purpose for which it was set. One of the things your doctor learned early on was the importance of budgeting time. (With the pressures of managed care, controlling a day's time has become more important than ever.) When you call for an appointment, the amount of time budgeted for your consultation or treatment will depend on the purpose for your visit. An hour appointment for a significant medical issue may be followed by three short follow-up visits, followed by a visit to the hospital to check on a patient. Thus, if you told the doctor you had one purpose, but come in with another, you may throw off the doctor's entire day. So, be polite. If you need more time with your doctor than originally planned, call ahead and rearrange your appointment (except, of course, in emergencies).

- Cancel appointments you cannot keep. This should be done at the earliest possible moment. Not only will it assist your doctor, but could be important to another of your doctor's patients who may have an urgent concern that needs to be "squeezed in."

- Be prepared to deal with the purpose of your appointment. As stated previously, when you come to your doctor's office, be prepared to deal with the matters at hand. In that way, a thirty-minute consultation won't end up taking an hour, leaving both you and your doctor struggling to catch up with the day.

- Even more important is respecting the doctor's "out of the office" time. Nothing irritates a doctor more than getting a weekend phone call from a patient who wants to discuss a problem he has had for several days. Do not expect a happy conversation if you call at midnight to report a problem that's been present since 8 AM. Do not call after hours to discuss matters about which the doctor can take no action until the next day (truly urgent or emergency matters excepted, of course). Finally, if you will need a refill of a prescription, do not wait until you take the last pill in the bottle before you call the doctor's office. To the doctor, that feels like the patient has jumped off a roof, shouting, "Catch me!" Not only is it hazardous for you—what if the doctor is out of the office and cannot be reached or you have trouble getting insurance approval—it is simply rude.

In short, follow the golden rule; be as considerate of your doctor's time as you want your doctor to be considerate of yours.

Have Reasonable Expectations

W e expect an awful lot from our doctors. Good bedside manners, twenty-four hour availability, warm stethoscopes, and a patient recovery rate of nearly 100 percent. Yet, in truth, while it is easy to get spoiled by medicine's daily successes, it is also unfair to expect continuous "miracles."

One common complaint of doctors is that their patients expect an accurate diagnosis and treatment regimen after the first visit. This certainly is not realistic. Proper diagnosis and treatment is often as much a ruling out as it is a ruling in. In pain control, proper treatment can be a matter of trying this and then trying that to come up with the optimal plan. So be a *patient* patient. Realize that your body is not a computer that will produce the desired result with a mere push of a button. If a reasonable time has passed and your pain is not adequately controlled, have a good talk with your doctor about it. If your doctor is unable to get a handle on treating your pain, it may be time to get a pain control specialist or a second opinion.

214

Even though this book is entitled *Power Over Pain,* it does not mean that all pain can always be absolutely eliminated. But it is rare indeed that pain cannot be controlled substantially. Still, there are some conditions in which just diminishing pain is the best that can be done, consistent with preventing untoward side effects. Sometimes, we have to adjust to difficult situations, and accept the truth of the old adage that a half a loaf is better than none. However, before you accept that your pain is just beyond the pale of total control, be sure you have been seen by a specialist and, if necessary, obtained a second opinion if the first specialist says that nothing better can be done.

Finding a Good Pain Control Doctor

Pain control, like other medical treatments, is a complex, sometimes maddening enterprise that, nonetheless, offers so much hope for so many people who currently feel that they are doomed to suffer for the rest of their lives. If your pain is to be treated, you cannot just open the Yellow Pages to the section on physicians, close your eyes, point and expect to find a good doctor. No, finding the right pain doctor does not occur by accident. You have to go about it the right way.

What are some of the methods to maximize your chances of finding a good pain doc? It isn't rocket science, but common sense. Here are some good sources:

- **Your own doctor.** Your doctor, as an involved medical professional, should know the good and bad doctors in the community, including pain control specialists. However, because of insurance issues or other matters, your doctor may be constrained from referring you to a specialist outside his or her medical group. So, if you're referred to a specialist within the same medical group, ask your doctor whether he or she would recommend this specialist to a close family member under the same circumstances. If not, ask for a referral to the specialist your doctor would recommend to a loved one. (That is assuming your insurance will cover the tab or you can afford to pay if it does not).

- **A friend who has suffered from a significant pain problem.** Word of mouth is a potent source of good doctors. If you have a friend who went to a pain specialist and was happy with the care, that doctor may be one you want to call your own.

- **The American Board of Pain Medicine.** This medical board maintains a list of doctors who are board certified in pain medicine. You can consult their web site, listed in the Appendix, to get the name of a certified physician near you.

- **Patient advocacy groups.** In many cities, there are support groups for people with AIDS, multiple sclerosis, fibromyalgia, etc. The assessment of the people in these groups concerning doctors they've dealt with is a particularly good source of information. The web site addresses of some of these groups may be found in the Appendix, too.

- **When all else fails, ask the librarian in your local public library.** A librarian's expertise is in knowing how to find out things.

The better your relationship with your doctor, the more likely your pain will be controlled. By expecting your rights as a patient to be honored by your doctor, and in turn, by doing your job as a patient, you will go a long way to assure that your pain will be controlled, allowing you to get on with the business of living.

CHAPTER 12

The Future of Pain Medicine

Medicine is undergoing a profound revolution that holds out great hope for the future of humankind. This is particularly true in the field of pain medicine. Already in development are novel treatments of pain that will give doctors more tools to help their patients. A few words about drug development will explain the process and give a hint of things to come.

If a mechanic wanted to improve the way a machine works, he would start by learning *how* it operates. Similarly, progress in treating pain requires us to learn how the pain system of the body works. We have already learned a lot about the physiology of the pain system, but there is much yet to discover. Laboratories all over the world are pursuing leads that will reveal even more about this marvelous system within us.

There are several new classes of drugs in development that seem likely to be major advances over currently available therapy. We'll give just three examples here.

When pain nerves are damaged, they send false signals to the spinal cord and brain. This leads to ongoing pain. One of the mechanisms by which this occurs has recently been discovered. The injured nerve manufactures too much of a "sodium channel" at the site of injury. Sodium channels are essential in the normal functioning of pain nerves. They allow the nerves to discharge, sending a signal to the brain. As you might imagine, too many sodium channels can translate to too many signals, and that means too much pain. The newly discovered sodium channel, dubbed the PN3 channel by researchers, is different in structure from the normal sodium channels

217

found in the brain and other parts of the body. In laboratory animals, drugs that specifically block the PN3 sodium channels dramatically reduce the amount of pain-related behavior the animals exhibit after nerve injury. Since the PN3 channel is not found in the brain or heart, drugs that specifically block it will be most unlikely to cause side effects on those organs. This would be a huge improvement, since the drugs we now have available block all types of sodium channels, not just the abnormal ones at sites of nerve damage. Now that we know a specific target in the nerve, there is a race on among pharmaceutical research companies to develop a drug that will specifically target this abnormality.

Remember the Chapter 2 discussion of neurotransmitters, those chemicals that carry pain signals from one nerve to another? One of them is called substance P. In order for substance P to elicit the appropriate response in the nerve cell to which it is carrying the message, that nerve must have a receptor into which the substance P can dock. That is called the substance P receptor (SPR). Not every cell in the body has SPR. In fact, in the spinal cord, SPR is found on only a minority of cells in the pain pathway. The cells that have SPR, however, seem to be particularly important in the transmission of severe, as opposed to mild, pain.

Some very clever researchers have linked a toxin called saporin to substance P. This two-link chain, or conjugate, may be likened to a guided missile, or, if you prefer a more classic metaphor, to a Trojan horse. When the substance P-saporin conjugate is injected into the spinal fluid of animals, the substance P part of the molecule causes it to bind to the substance P receptor on the surface of the cells committed to transmitting severe pain information. After the substance P binds to the receptor, the whole conjugate is taken into the cell. There, the toxin, which is otherwise unable to enter and damage the cell, is able to kill the cell. Thus, only cells bearing the SPR on their surface are destroyed. The consequence? Within days after the injection, the animals that have been used in the development of this potential elixir

218

exhibit a dramatically lower response to painful stimuli, but seem otherwise intact. This drug is currently under development with the hope that it will prove to be a single injection to relieve pain in cancer patients. Imagine the possibilities: tremendous control over pain with few, if any, significant side effects.

The third exciting development on the horizon is a modification of opioid therapy. As you know by now, close to two hundred years after the development of morphine, opioids remain the most useful and powerful medicines for a wide variety of painful conditions. Yet they are not without their shortcomings. Physical dependence is a side effect that requires management, and tolerance sometimes limits their benefit. A new class of drug now in development may yield the benefit of opioids without these problems.

You'll recall that opioids exert their beneficial effect at the synapse, that small gap between contiguous neurons where chemicals secreted by one cell can affect the behavior of the other cell. Did you ever wonder what turns off the action of a neurotransmitter? That is, once the chemical is in the synapse, why doesn't it just keep on exerting its effect endlessly?

It turns out that there are a number of mechanisms to prevent this from happening. For some neurotransmitters, the chemical is actively taken up by the very cell that first secreted it. There it is repackaged for subsequent use. You might call it the neuron's recycling program.

Other neurotransmitters are rapidly destroyed by enzymes normally present in the synapse. For example, there is a class of enzymes called enkephalinases that naturally degrade the opioid in the synapse. This limits the duration of their activity in the synapse.

What would happen if the activity of the enkephalinases were inhibited? One would predict that either naturally occurring opioids (such as the endorphins and enkephalins) or the medical forms of opioids (such as morphine) would persist in the synapse for a longer period of time. One would also predict that the longer persistence of the opioid in the synapse would lead to a greater pain reduction. In fact, that is exactly what happens. In animal models, enkephalinase inhibitors are powerful pain relievers, equivalent to opioids. What is more, in animals, at least, they are not associated with the problems of tolerance or dependence. By themselves they are powerful pain relievers, and it is likely that enkephalinase inhibitors would dramatically enhance the pain relieving capability of administered opioids. At the time of the writing of this book, human trials of enkephalinase inhibitors have just begun.

———————■———————

Pain, like death and taxes, will always be with us. But, unlike death and taxes, pain can be effectively alleviated or even eliminated. We need not meekly accept its awful reign that Albert Schweitzer described as the terrible lord of mankind. We hope this book has been helpful to you, and that, with its assistance, you and your doctor can truly exercise power over pain.

Appendix

Appendix

The purpose of this appendix is to give you sources of further information and assistance. While we have tried to select only reliable sources, you must recognize that we are not responsible for, nor do we necessarily endorse, everything you will find from these sources. For your convenience, we plan to make available links to the web sites listed below (and new ones that may become available after the publication of this book) at our publisher's web site, www.internationaltaskforce.org.

General Pain Support

American Chronic Pain Assn.
PO Box 850
Rocklin, CA 95677
(916) 632-0922
www.theacpa.org

American Pain Foundation
111 South Calvert Street
Suite 2700
Baltimore, MD 21202
www.painfoundation.com

Joint Commission on the Accreditation of Healthcare Organizations (JCAHO)
One Renaissance Boulevard,
Oakbrook Terrace, IL 60181
(630) 792-5000
www.jcaho.org

Mayday Pain Project
www.painandhealth.org

Pain.com
www.pain.com

Professional Organizations

American Academy of Pain Management
13947 Mono Way #A
Sonora, CA 95370
(209) 533-9744
www.aapainmanage.org

American Pain Society
4700 West Lake Avenue
Glenview, IL 60025
(847) 375-4715
www.ampainsoc.org

Professional Organizations (cont.)

American Academy of Pain Medicine
4700 West Lake Avenue
Glenview, IL 60025
(847) 375-4731
www.painmed.org

American Academy of Orofacial Pain
19 Mantua Road
Mount Royal, NJ 08061
(856) 423-3629
www.aaop.org

International Association for the Study of Pain
909 NE 43rd Street
Suite 306
Seattle, WA 98105-6020
(206) 547-6409
www.iasp-pain.org

Hospice and End-of-Life Information

National Hospice and Palliative Care Organization
1700 Diagonal Road
Suite 300
Alexandria, VA 22314
(703) 516-4928
www.nhpco.org

Hospice Education Institute
190 Westbrook Road
Essex, CT 06426-1510
(860) 767-1620
www.hospiceworld.org

International Task Force on Euthanasia and Assisted Suicide
P.O. Box 760
Steubenville, OH 43952
(740) 282-3810
(800) 958-5678
www.internationaltaskforce.org

Diseases and Conditions

Arthritis Foundation
1330 West Peachtree Street
Atlanta, GA 30309
(800) 2283-7800
www.arthritis.org

Fibromyalgia Network
P.O. Box 31750
Tucson, AZ 85751
(800) 853-2929
www.fmnetnews.com

Interstitial Cystitis Association
51 Monroe Street - Suite 1402
Rockville, MD 20850
(301) 610-5300
www.ichelp.org

National Cancer Institute
Public Inquiries Office
Building 31 , Room 10A03
31 Center Drive
MSC 2580
Bethesda MD 20892-2580
(301) 435-3848
www.cancernet.nci.nih.gov

National Spinal Cord Injury Association
8701 Georgia Ave., Suite 500
Silver Spring, MD 20910
(800) 962-9629
www.spinalcord.org

Endometriosis Association
8585 North 76th Place
Milwaukee, WI 53223
(414) 355-2200
www.endometriosisassn.org

International Pelvic Pain Society
Women's Medical Plaza
2006 Brookwood Medical
Center Dr., Suite 402
Birmingham, AL 35209
www.pelvicpain.org

National Multiple Sclerosis Society
733 Third Avenue
New York, NY 10017
(800-344-4867)

National Vulvodynia Association
Box 4491
Silver Spring, MD 20914-4491
(301) 299-0775
www.nva.org

National Headache Foundation
428 W. St. James Place
2nd Floor
Chicago, IL 60614-2750
(888) NHF-5552
www.headaches.org

Diseases and Conditions (cont.)

National Organization for Rare Disorders
P.O. Box 8923
New Fairfield, CT 06812-8923
(203) 746-6518
www.rarediseases.org

Reflex Sympathetic Dystrophy Syndrome (RSD) Association of America
P.O. Box 821
Haddonfield, NJ 08033
(856) 795-8845
www.rsds.org

Vulvar Pain Foundation
P.O. Box 177
Graham, NC 27253
(336) 226-0704
www.vulvarpainfoundation.org

Trigeminal Neuralgia Association
P.O. Box 340
Barnegat Light, NJ 08006
(609) 361-6250
www.tna-support.org

Sickle Cell Disease Association of America
200 Corporate Point
Suite 495
Culver City, CA 90230-7633
(800) 421-8453
www.sicklecelldisease.org

Advance Health Care Directive

For more information on the Protective Medical Decisions Document (PMDD), a Durable Power of Attorney for Health Care, contact:

International Task Force
P.O. Box 760
Steubenville, Ohio 43952 USA
(800) 958-5678

Index

Index

New York Post, Detroit News, San Diego Union Tribune, Sacramento Bee, and the *Cleveland Plain Dealer,* among many others. Smith authored the chapter on assisted suicide for *The Encyclopedia of Crime and Justice* and an article on the topic in Microsoft's on-line encyclopedia, *Encarta.*

Smith is the author of numerous books, including *Forced Exit: The Slippery Slope from Assisted Suicide to Legalized Murder* (Times Books, 1997), a broad-based exposé of the assisted-suicide/euthanasia movement. His most recent book, *Culture of Death: The Assault on Medical Ethics in America* (Encounter Books, 2001), is a warning about the dangers of the modern bioethics movement. *Culture of Death* was named One of the Ten Outstanding Books of the Year and Best Health Book of the Year for 2001 (Independent Publisher Book Awards).

Smith has appeared on more than 900 television or radio talk/interview programs, including such national programs as *ABC Nightline, Good Morning America, Larry King Live, CNN Crossfire, CNN World Report, CBS Evening News,* and *CNN Talk Back Live.* He has also appeared internationally on *Voice of America, CNN International,* and on programs originating in Great Britain (BBC), Australia, New Zealand, and Canada.

Smith lives in Oakland, California, with his wife, syndicated columnist Debra J. Saunders.

———————————■———————————